Mental Handicap

Facilitating Holistic Care

USING NURSING MODELS SERIES

General Editors:

Susan E Norman SRN, DNCERT, RNT
Senior Tutor, The Nightingale School, St Thomas's Hospital, London
Computer Assisted Learning (CAL) Project Leader

Jane E Schober SRN, RCNT, DipN Ed, DipN (Lond), RNT
Lecturer, Nursing Studies, Institute of Advanced Nursing Education,
Royal College of Nursing

Christine Webb BA, MSc, PhD, SRN, RSCN, RNT
Principal Lecturer in Nursing, Department of Nursing, Health and
Applied Social Studies, Bristol Polytechnic, Bristol

The views expressed in this book are those of the authors of individual chapters
and do not necessarily reflect the opinions of the series editors.

Mental Handicap
Facilitating Holistic Care

Paul Barber

MSc, BA, SRN, RMN, RNMS, RNT

Specialist Lecturer, Institute of Advanced Nursing Education,
Royal College of Nursing

HODDER AND STOUGHTON
LONDON SYDNEY AUCKLAND TORONTO

British Library Cataloguing in Publication Data

Barber, Paul
    Mental handicap: facilitating holistic
    care.——(Using nursing models).
    1. Mentally handicapped——Care and
    treatment
    I. Title   II. Series
    362.3'8   HV3004

    ISBN 0 340 36999 X

First published 1987

Typeset by Macmillan India Ltd., Bangalore 560 025

Printed in Great Britain
for Hodder and Stoughton Educational,
a division of Hodder and Stoughton Ltd.,
Mill Road, Dunton Green, Sevenoaks, Kent TNYD
by The Eastern Press Ltd., London and Reading

Table of Contents

List of Contributors

John Aldridge RNMH, RMN, RCNT began his nursing career at Park Prewett Hospital, Basingstoke, qualifying as RMN, before undertaking a post-registration course at Borocourt Hospital, Reading, and obtaining his RNMS. He worked on the Mary Sheridan Unit at the above hospital as Charge Nurse where he came into contact with clients suffering multiple handicaps. While there he developed an awareness of the need to involve the family of clients in care, and 'family therapy' has since become a central theme in his work. In 1980 he moved to Princess Marina Hospital, Northampton, as a nurse teacher, where he has been involved in formulating a nursing model for use in Mental Handicap nursing.

Paul Barber MSc, BA, RNT, RNMS, RMN, SRN trained in the late sixties as a psychiatric nurse in mental handicap and mental illness, later qualifying as a General Nurse. He worked as a Charge Nurse in an infirmary and assessment area for mentally handicapped adults prior to appointment as a Charge Nurse with group-work responsibilities in acute psychiatry. He gained a Social Science degree from the Open University in 1974, and commenced postgraduate studies in Nursing Education and Administration at Edinburgh University in 1976, which allowed registration as a Nurse Tutor. He was employed as a Psychiatric Nurse Tutor in 1976 and a Senior Tutor for Mental Illness and Mental Handicap in 1978. Paul Barber has been a Specialist Lecturer within the Institute of Advanced Nursing Education at the Royal College of Nursing since 1982, where he teaches personal and professional development, experiential learning strategies, counselling, group work and therapeutic community practice. He was a member of the working party—and contributor—to the ENB learning package *Caring for People with Mental Handicap*. He is currently researching the implications of group work and personal growth for education and undergoing advanced training as a Gestalt Therapist.

Martin Brown RMN, RCNT, RNT, CERTIFICATE IN ADULT BEHAVIOURAL PSYCHOTHERAPY, DIPN ED is currently the Director of Nursing Services, Tooting Bec Hospital. He was recently Assistant Nurse Advisor in Mental Handicap and Mental Illness in the Department of Nursing Policy and Practice at the Royal College of Nursing. He originally trained at Banstead Hospital in the late sixties and has worked in a variety of clinical settings including the community. He was employed as a Community Nurse in the Hounslow area before undertaking training in behaviour therapy at the Maudsley Hospital. Martin Brown furthered his experience by working for two years as a Nurse Therapist, spent the subsequent year researching behaviour therapy in primary care, and returned to the Maudsley Hospital as Course Tutor of the Behaviour Therapy course.

Amanda Gunner RNMH, DIPN (LOND), CERT ED, RNT nursed within a variety of settings, including hospital, hostel and community environments after qualifying as a RNMH. Whilst employed as a Sister at Hilda Lewis House, Croydon, she developed an interest in education that was carried into her later rôle as a sister with Croydon's Community Mental Handicap Team. She was a tutor in St Lawrence's Hospital, Caterham and secretary to the Tutors' Interest Group within the Society of Mental Handicap Nursing of the Royal College of Nursing. Recently she has taken up the post of Senior Tutor with the Waltham Forest Health Authority.

Ian Norman BA (HONS), MSc, RNMS, RMN, RGN, CQSW qualified as a Registered Nurse for Mental Handicap and Mental Illness in 1976, working with clients from mental handicap before entering Keele University to read for a degree in Social Science and qualifying professionally as a social worker. He worked as a Probation Officer in Greater London before returning to nursing and undertaking RGN training. He gained an MSc in Nursing Education from the University of Edinburgh and is currently Nurse Tutor at West Park Hospital, Epsom.

Margaret Williams RNMS, RGN, RNT, DipN (LOND), CERT ED, BEd (HONS), MA (PSYCHOLOGY OF MENTAL HANDICAP) trained initially at Stoke Park Hospital, Bristol, for the qualification of RNMS and at Bristol Royal Infirmary for her SRN, and followed this by working with clients from differing dependency groups. In 1972 she opened a rehabilitation ward at Purdown Hospital, Bristol, introducing individual training programmes there. In 1975 she qualified as Registered Nurse Tutor, becoming Senior Nurse Tutor at Stoke Park Hospital the following year. She has acted as examiner for the English National Board and was a contributor to the ENB Publication *Caring for People with Mental Handicap*. Currently, she is employed as Education Officer (Mental Handicap) with the English National Board.

Foreword

This is a book for nurses who already know about holistic nursing, know about mentally handicapped people, but who need help to achieve a holistic approach to the care of their clients.

They will obtain such help from this book, whether they work in hospital or in the community, in clinical practice or in management. Furthermore, they will gain comfort from the recognition of their need for support and of their role in the supervision of other staff.

At a time when books for beginners proliferate, it is good to find here one which credits readers with already possessing knowledge, with motivation for progressing, with the ability to think deeply and with the capacity for a creative approach to their practice.

In work with the mentally handicapped, the application of theories and models is not an easy task. The authors have here succeeded in facilitating an approach to the process of nursing by demonstrating how a critical analysis of existing models and a judicious selection from them can benefit patient care. Their use of examples from their own practice shows that they are concerned with real life, not with remote theories.

The authors are to be congratulated on the way this book promotes creativity and encourages the reader to approach any task with confidence.

Annie T Altschul
CBE, BA (Hons) London, BA (Hons) Open University, MSc, FRCN, RGN, RMN, RNT
Emeritus Professor of Nursing Studies
University of Edinburgh

Introduction

Nursing care for people who suffer mental handicap has come a long way; it still has a long way to go. The purpose of this book is to stimulate you into taking it further. This book does not seek to provide polished water-tight accounts, of how to use 'nursing theory' or to fuel further academic debate as to 'the nature of nursing'. If you want firm answers to these issues you will need to look elsewhere. What we attempt in the following pages is to share those approaches to care which we have found useful in order to rationalise, communicate and understand what it is we do. We hope to share with you our doubts, the questioning process we bring to our work, our failures and success. We do not have authoritative answers—nor do we endeavour to seek these out—for our exploration is ongoing. A word of caution though, we do have our biases; we believe that social interaction—especially when of an educative nature—and relationship skills underpin much of care; that 'theories of nursing' help to provide the carer with a 'cognitive map' and that 'models of nursing' may act as catalysts in the creation of care programmes to suit the unique demands of individual clients.

Nursing models are here perceived as tools of enquiry rather than answers to problems, and are taken to be a 'means' rather than the 'end' to which we work.

Attached to each chapter is a Summary orientating the reader to those issues it unfolds; at the end of each chapter a Critique examines any inconsistencies of argument. This is followed by a list of Salient Questions to reflect upon, and it is here that readers may ponder out for themselves such issues as the 'nature of nursing' and the 'gains and costs of using nursing models'.

Specifically, nursing models are suggested to enhance the development of facilitation skills (Chapter 1), community nursing (Chapter 2), clinical practice (Chapter 3), behaviour therapy (Chapter 4), service management (Chapter 5) and staff supervision and development (Chapter 6).

To summarise, this book attempts to stimulate you—the reader—to reflect upon 'how you care', 'how you may further the care you provide' and 'how you can develop within yourself interpersonal and perceptive qualities' that increase your potential as a therapeutic agent.

Paul Barber
Royal College of Nursing, 1987

I

Preparing the way for nursing models: the nurse's role as a process facilitator— an educational perspective

Paul Barber

Summary
In the first of our chapters addressing the uses of nursing models, stresses are explored which detract from the benefits of a nursing-process approach to care. One such stress is seen to be the tendency to 'control' patients in contrast to 'caring' for them. Facilitation to health is advocated to prevent this, where the nurse functions as a resource person who educates the client to self-help skills. It is suggested that nursing models are enriched by this strategy, for their underlying rationale of holistic care complements a nurse-facilitation rôle where the self-awareness of both nurse and client may be enhanced and directed towards therapeutic goals. Finally, styles of intervention are discussed and comparisons made between 'authoritative' and 'facilitative' modes of relating. Eight models of nursing are selected for appraisal, with regard to their view of clients, nursing action and health.

Paul Barber

Introduction

It has long been recognised that most of the stress endemic to nursing focuses within the profession's interpersonal relationships. You find relationship stresses in peer group dialogue, inter-professional discussion, and most of all in the nurse–patient relationship. This latter area in the domain of mental handicap is even more fraught, for our clients are less amenable to treatment, may be hyperactive, have anti-social habits or be profoundly impoverished in their communication. An inner sense of well-being is essential for a nurse

exposed to such pressure but any resemblance of composure is under constant attack from the demands of bureaucratic managers and nurse educationalists who teach a reality very different from everyday clinical practice.

(Barber, 1986)

When nurses have no identifiable perspective or model of care to work from, the pressures described above crowd in and generate confusion. This confusion combines with a sense of loss of purpose causing them to be at the mercy of whatever framework is available to offer support. It is as well to remember just what is the nature of the stress that nurses bear:

The situations likely to evoke stress in nurses are familiar. Nurses are in constant contact with people who are physically ill or injured, often seriously. The recovery of patients is not certain and will not always be complete. Nursing patients who have incurable diseases is one of the nurse's most distressing tasks. Nurses are confronted with the threat and the reality of suffering and death as few lay people are. Their work involves carrying out tasks which, by ordinary standards are distasteful, disgusting, and frightening. Intimate physical contact with patients arouses strong libidinal and erotic wishes and impulses that may be difficult to control. The work situation arouses very strong and mixed feeling in the nurse: pity, compassion, and love, guilt and anxiety; hatred and resentment of the care given to the patient.

(Menzies, 1960)

All this is heavy enough for anyone, yet when you consider the lack of counselling within the profession and dearth of leadership, it seems natural enough that nurses let routines do their thinking for them and structure their clinical performance to fend off further anxiety.

Examples of how nurses have structured their activities in an effort to fight interpersonal stress are shown in Figure 1.1 alongside the consequences these have on professional culture.

In such an environment, where psychological defences are rife, nursing becomes mechanistic and instrumental, and may end up treating its clients as intruders who threaten successful staff performance and composure.

Nursing process and the promise of 'change'

Traditionally, nursing has evolved in the shadow of medicine and adopted a similar 'authoritative' approach to care. Patients, who are already isolated behind hospital walls, were until com-

paratively recently further estranged from themselves and their potential social reality by nurses who assumed responsibility for them on their behalf. When nurses take custody of 'patients' in this way, nursing care treads a path close to 'social control'. When nurses act as agents of control, they run the risk of perpetuating those very behaviours they seek to correct therapeutically, namely dependence, depersonalisation and regression. Such behaviours, when encouraged by nurses, lead to the syndrome of learned helplessness known as institutionalisation.

All this is frustrating enough in the care of those who—as you and I—live an independent life and can return to an external community, but in the care of mentally handicapped people such effects are devastating, for we abet dependence upon the institution to the extent that it can become total and destroy initiative. Nursing such as this may produce effects which are far graver than those conditions it attempts to relieve.

Fig. 1.1   Social defences common to nursing (after Menzies, 1960)

Social defences	Examples and Consequences
Splitting up of nurse–patient relationship	Task fixation; treating all patients alike; listing duties; restriction of one-to-one relationships; nurse–patient friendships strongly discouraged
Depersonalisation and categorisation	Patients seen as conditions; uniformity of management, performance and attitude seen as preferable to individuality or creativity of approach
Denial of feelings	Staff expected to control their own feelings and show no emotion; involvement feared; control replaces care
Ritual task performance	Anxiety of free choice reduced by systems of instrumental activity and nursing procedures; decisions shelved until new procedures produced or policies formed; questioning discouraged
Avoidance of decisions	Decisions pushed upwards to senior managers or medics; blame pushed downwards onto juniors; rôle-blurring
Avoidance of change	Full consent of everyone sought before change can take place; progress only as fast as slowest team member; fear of facing new situations because of need to restructure existing defences
Checks and counter-checks	Everything has a tendency to be obsessionally recorded; trust of others and their skills a rarity; fear of failure a constant concern

Many unhealthy characteristics have arisen in nursing care and remain because nurse educators and practitioners have been unable to challenge the traditional 'medical–custodial model of care' with a more meaningful one. All this has now changed, for in this book alone some half dozen models of care are discussed. We no longer have any excuse for burying our heads in the sand and leaving it all to fate.

Although—very simply—the nursing process may be reduced to a clerking duty that lists problems and provides a check-list of things for nurses to do, when it is fully utilised and meaningfully applied it provides an impetus for movement away from the routines and defensive gameplay described by Menzies (1960).

Consider, for example, a definition of the nursing process as offered by the World Health Organization:

> The nursing process is a term applied to a system of characteristic nursing interventions in the care of individuals, families and/or communities. In detail it involves the use of scientific methods for identifying the needs of the patient/client/family or community and for using these to select those

which can most effectively be met by nursing care; it also includes planning to meet these needs, provide the care and evaluate the results . . . defines objectives, sets priorities, identifies care to be given and mobilises resources . . . The information feedback from evaluation of outcome should initiate desirable changes in subsequent interventions in similar nursing care situations. In this way, nursing becomes a dynamic process lending itself to adaption and improvement.

(WHO Document 5.8.77)

There is nothing too daunting in the above; the nurse sets about identifying the client's needs, plans interventions to meet them, implements strategies thought to be appropriate and evaluates the effect of this within the ever-changing care picture. As to how to go about the above, well, there is an abundance of nursing models to help us. With regard to the above, the 'process' appears to be a socially interactive one closely associated with the concept of 'holistic care', where the total needs of a person are considered and the defences described by Menzies redressed.

Figure 1.2 illustrates in simple terms the 'humanistic' rationale underpinning holistic care

Fig. 1.2   Influences underpinning the concept of holistic care

Individual needs	Care objectives	Necessary nursing qualities and skills
Psychological needs	Personal security Understanding of one's own inner states Self-esteem needs Sense of purpose and meaning Achieving as full potential as possible Self-sufficiency	For nurses to have achieved as fully as they are able the previous psychological care objectives for themselves, and to value personal growth and the acquisition of empathy and counselling skills
Social needs	Security of expression and communication Acceptance by others A sense of belonging Interpersonal sensitivity Independence	For nurses to have achieved to a sufficient degree the previous social objectives for themselves, plus skills in assertion and relationship management, and the ability to teach the same
Physiological needs	Freedom from discomfort The meeting of dietary and hygiene needs Physical exercise Skills in self-maintenance	For nurses to be physically healthy; able to employ specialist medical management, knowledge and skills

and gives examples of what care objectives ensue and how they in turn make requirements of the nurse.

The 'nursing process' provides a framework where a client can be facilitated to health rather than controlled as a patient and viewed as the passive recipient of a disease. The nursing vision is broadened, adopts the stance of holistic care (Figure 1.2) and encourages nurses to see themselves as 'resource people' who humanise care and translate the formal demands of specialist approaches—such as medicine, psychology and the science of psychiatry—into warm individual terms.

The status of the nurse is secondary in the above climate to rôle efficiency, and the nurse may become more a friend without feeling that they are stepping out of rôle. Here carer and cared-for share in a therapeutic environment where mutual effort is directed towards the resolution of shared problems.

Central to this approach is the nurse's ability to mobilise the client's own self-enabling skills; they no longer dictate 'authoritative care', but rather liberate their potential as socially dynamic and therapeutic agents.

The nurse as a facilitator

Facilitation does not set itself up to replace, remove, or compete with other models of care, but rather to use the best of each approach to meet the needs of individual clients.

As facilitators, nurses retain their existing knowledge base but use it differently, in that they more clearly attend to the social significance of their actions. When personal qualities are invested in clinical and professional practice, care becomes warm rather than remote and person management moves towards goals which are open and shared; the ward becoming tailored to the needs of the client rather than he to its routines.

As a facilitator the nurse comes of age and gains interactive integrity; genuine depth of feeling may be placed in the frame of nursing practice in the shape of empathic understanding and that openness that attends therapeutic coun-

selling. Nurses gain responsibility for 'themselves' along with others; facilitation allows a diversity of purpose to exist, is able to initiate sharing, and can avoid the defensive game-play that is enacted to protect bureaucratic rules. Nurses may therefore concentrate upon developing themselves and their clients in the way of creative and spontaneous adaptation.

Although nursing has evolved many ways with which to meet the physiological and medical needs of its clients, it has only paid lip-service— for the main part—to its interpersonal rôle. In consequence, nurses tend to feel more secure when dealing with medical needs than in the use or enhancement of social skills.

Medical needs may be easily reduced to systematic tasks. Interpersonal and social intervention skills—by contrast—require acknowledgement of the social and personal processes involved plus such qualities as the ability to risk checking things out, and side-stepping defensive staff–client collusions.

When taken to extremes, 'process dead' and task-fixated vision produces nursing which cares more for the formal institutional system than the person. If mere tasks are performed without consideration of the social processes involved, more care is lavished on managerial maintenance than people. In hospital terms, the ward is nursed rather than its patients.

This is not without cautionary humour: the ward would be a marvellous place if it weren't for the patients! The isolation of instrumental activity from its social perspective may give operational success but fails to provide care. A practical example is as follows: We may fulfil the simple 'task' of carrying out the medicine round —in that medication is taken by our residents— but cause the individuals to feel so undervalued or in the way that they are unable to break into our routine and voice their anxiety regarding the medicine they take. At the first opportunity the resident goes to the toilet and spits out his tablets. If these are anti-convulsants, dire results may ensue, from fitting to status epilepticus. In the field of mental handicap this may arise from the simplest of causes; perhaps the client's medication was recently altered and the new tablets tasted unpleasant—easy enough to remedy; the point is, attention to the social 'process' is just as important as doing 'tasks'.

Much of nursing care—and its management—is intuitive and runs the risk of appearing superficial, abstract or undefined. Many nurses therefore become uncertain as to why they are working, how to transmit to others the rationale which they work, or to conceptualise just what senior staff expect of them. Models of nursing can help to clarify the above, but certain interpersonal awarenesses and skills are demanded of the nurse if these are to be used in a credible therapeutic fashion.

My own bias here is my belief that nurses will need to accept the philosophy of 'care facilitation' and 'personal growth' if they are to use nursing models fruitfully. Taking Menzies' (1960) observations of nursing's interpersonal malfunction, i.e.

> depersonalisation; categorisation; the denial of individualisation; emotional detachment; splitting-up of the nurse–patient relationship; pushing of blame downwards and responsibility upwards; and ritualistic adherence;

we have ample evidence of what must be left behind if we are to liberate our energies for creative care. If these symptoms of our 'professional neurosis' remain unchecked, for any one step we take forward towards 'person sensitivity' we will need to take two steps back again to pay homage to 'the system'.

Carl Rogers (1983) has discovered much to enable our understanding of what we must work towards to achieve 'person centred' professional relationships. Rogers' propositions regarding the outcomes of the person-valuing process serve as guides to the direction we must move to rectify our 'institutional vision', those ethics we need to adopt for such a function and what qualities care facilitators should value.

Figure 1.3 lists those qualities Rogers sees as evolving from an individual's movement in the direction of increased growth and maturity. Applying these insights to nurse-to-nurse relationships—or interprofessional dialogue—the following 'process strengthening' guidelines are suggested for peer relating.

Don't seek to just restrict experience—keeping the lid upon a boiling pot—but give others the chance and time to verbalise or express their stresses and listen accordingly.

Shape conversation in such a way as it becomes purposeful—state your intentions and request feedback and check things out, rather than using conversation as social lubricant or flight away from the present.

Encourage colleagues to express their fears, anxieties and opinions—so that you may both know them and support them more. If you don't care for your staff, how may they in turn care for the residents? You are an effective rôle model and

Fig. 1.3 Consequences of person valuing and self-aware practice/qualities for facilitators to develop (adapted from Rogers, 1983)

Movement away from	Façades, pretence, and putting up a front
	Rigid concepts of 'what ought to be'
	Meeting the expectations of others for the sake of 'having to please'
Gaining greater	Self-direction and valuing the same in others
	Positive feelings towards oneself and tolerance of personal failings
	Sensitivity to others and acceptance of them
Less need to	Hold onto tried and tested routines in preference to exploring new potentialities
	Pretend and hide real feelings
Valuing more	Deep, honest and communicative relationships
	The ability to be open and aware of one's own inner reactions and feelings and sensitive to external events

need to relay care in your relationships with them.

Display pleasant receptiveness—don't gripe about your lot; a cheerful approach will often solicit information otherwise left unsaid. Try not to make the care climate too heavy or serious, so causing fears of criticism or punishment to replace the joys of sharing.

Be prepared to earn your colleagues' respect through 'what you do' rather than the 'rank or status' you hold—accept your rôle of culture carrier, and share your problems rather than hide them to protect your rank.

Pay attention to your own interpersonal defences— i.e. a rigid denial of problems which may obstruct your communication. Ask for feedback; what do others 'like least' and 'like best' about your style of work?

Accept your own fallibility—be prepared to make mistakes and face up to them having once made them: even share them so you and others may learn together.

Don't be afraid to clarify the meaning of a remark—establish that both you and the person to whom you relate share a similar interpretation. Misinterpretation is the commonest cause of frustration, anger and poor interpersonal relations.

The above aims de-ritualise and break into collusive staff networks that may develop; they also give pointers for the development of a self-actualising climate where nurses may—against all previous odds and the wildest pipe-dreams— start to care for themselves and each other! Professional, personal and therapeutic growth may then occur simultaneously. The inculcation of self-awareness so stimulated by the above objectives acts as a catalyst of personal development. True care transcends instrumental activity and mere rôle performance.

Relating Rogers' criteria to 'client-centred therapy' the following facilitator intentions seem consistent with 'process-alive care' in respect of nurse–client relating:

Be aware that 'residents' watch and remember nurses' actions and use them as examples and standards for ward behaviour—in this context you carry the culture of your ward, and are the most potent of 'behaviour modifiers' open to clients.

Don't force residents into activities—rather suggest. Guide more than direct; give space and freedom to discuss and reflect on the alternatives of an action.

Realise that the individual before you is experiencing a situation she perceives as both serious and meaningful—all too often you may forget the intense effort a client needs to generate in order to perform a task, which you consider easy.

Reward all positive action—no matter how trivial, with a word or smile so as to shape desired behaviour responses. This is the essence of care and the positive use of the 'nurse–client' relationship.

Approach your residents as individuals—conveying an interest in them as valued persons distinct from either status or rôle. Second-class citizenship has no place in a therapeutic setting.

Observe and listen before entering into an ongoing interaction—and once involved listen attentively. Intuitive timing may develop from so simple a start.

Deal openly and honestly with your clients—if they ask questions which are confidential to their own or another's situation, say that you feel the area to be confidential. Never make an excuse or mislead. It is just as easy to state your 'concerns' as to avoid giving reasons; if something is not in your power to reveal, say so.

Be alert to changes in posture—tone of voice and mood. Fit in your own remarks and emotional tone accordingly.

Be aware of your own effect on a person's behaviour—to isolate oneself from a social interaction is to deny your own effect upon another's behaviour, and leads to unbalanced observation and reporting.

The above aims seek to enhance 'process' vision. They address the social process rather than the end product—or task—for which you work; in this they are qualitative and look at what is happening now between people. Being aware of the 'here and now' reality of care provision prevents you from flying away into a routine frame of mind where you can turn off until the procedure is over-and-done-with. Being 'really there' for the clients you are with is an integral component of 'true' care; anything else is a sham and does not deserve the label of 'care'.

The above list may similarly be appreciated as suggesting what makes for ethical interpersonal practice. It is in no way exhaustive but only a guide from which you may generate your own code of practice.

Therapeutic interventions: becoming aware of the options

Facilitation in relation to nursing implies a socially aware style of care where the nurse acts as a co-ordinator of interpersonal, clinical and managerial resource, from whence skills are derived to mobilise the client's capacity for self-directed and stress-free living. Those energies previously employed to control the patient and protect the bureaucracy of the hospital can now be released to develop the potential of nurse–client interaction. This increases the nurses' therapeutic currency.

When nurses act as guardians of a ward—and formal systems of care—they are drawn into interventions which are predominately 'parenting', that is to say their interventions may be exclusively of the following nature:

(1) **Directive**: judgemental and critical, seeking to direct the client's behaviour.
(2) **Informative**: instructs and interprets for the client, relays information.
(3) **Confronting**: challenges the attitudes, beliefs and behaviours of the client.

The above are often delivered in authoritarian ways which rob them of their therapeutic potential. Used well, such interventions help to provide a framework and shape to the nurse–patient relationship. These modes of response may be compared to nurturing when the nurse acts as a figure who functions as an extension of the client's conscience, confronts him with reality or informs him of the options open to him.

Used therapeutically, authoritative interventions such as the above are value-free, but when nurses limit themselves to their sole use a restrictive environment may arise which interferes with the development of the client's own self-enabling skills.

Directive interventions are relevant to the delegation of responsibilities and tasks. They are necessary when the facilitator must assume an autocratic style of operation rather than a consensual one, for instance in times of emergency or crisis. Similarly, *informative* interventions are useful to convey new insight, meaning and knowledge. *Confronting* interventions may also be used positively to identify restrictive attitudes and behaviours and to introduce these into the client's awareness.

We must be alert to the attachment of moral correctness or judgemental opinions of 'right-and-wrong' to authoritative interventions. They are simply tools with relevance to specific situations.

As facilitators nurses retain relevant use of the earlier interventions as part of their therapeutic arsenal while extending their range to include the following self-enabling ones:

(4) **Releasing**: these aim to relieve tensions in the client, encourage his laughing, crying or need to vent anger. Here a climate is created to enable the expression and discharge of disabling emotion.
(5) **Reflective**: facilitates the reflection necessary for the production of self-insight and the enactment of self-directed learning; guides the client towards the resolution of his own problems and hence greater independence.
(6) **Supportive**: confirms the intrinsic value of the client and his worth as an individual.

Applying facilitation

The art of successful facilitation requires nurses to develop further their degree of self- and social-awareness, plus intuition as to which intervention to use and a feeling for when and how to use it.

On meeting a situation where caring interventions may be made, a facilitator needs to decide if the objectives of care would be furthered by professional intrusion. Much of a therapeutic nature can occur without an obvious intervention and be the more valid in being client-directed and spontaneous. Knowing when to withhold from action, to listen and observe with free and open attention, or just to share silence with a client is as significant a care skill as to intervene.

Having decided to intervene the nurse needs to ask 'which is the most appropriate intervention to make?' Initially an authoritarian intervention may be selected to frame a mutually productive climate for exchange. No one intervention will be all sufficient in itself; interventions will flow one to another as new awarenesses unfold. The nurse will need to stay open and alert as to the next intervention to make.

As greater rapport with the process develops, facilitative intervention will be suggested.

Any one intervention is valuable only insofar as it stimulates self-enablement. The facilitator needs to therefore aim at being *directive* to the extent that it stimulates the self-direction of his client; *informative* to the degree that it generates the client's own interpretations; *confronting* to the level the client is able to solicit his own confrontation; *releasing* to the point that the client is able to select and manage his own tension-releasing behaviour; *reflective* to the degree that it induces the client to develop on his own responses and find a personal answer: and *supportive* to the stage of orientating the client to an awareness of his own worthiness.

As to other qualities, these are dependent on the richness of the nurse's own humanity, and regard for others who share the human condition.

> Your medicine is in you, and you do not observe it. Your ailment is from yourself, and you do not register it.
>
> (Sabistari)

Choosing a model: a walk through the market place

It was earlier stated that nurses had a duty to familiarise themselves with the range of nursing models at their disposal; for from these a rationale may be chosen for caring interventions. We have examined the practice of facilitation where nurses may use their own personal qualities and social skills to enrich the development of clients. Nurses were seen as stimulators of personal growth besides being maintainers of health and survival.

As a resource person, the nurse acts as a guide who steers clients through life's challenges and supports them in times of decision. Nursing models provide a framework for this exchange, but it is wise to select one with which you are in affinity. For instance, if you personally approach the giving of care in a predominantly sociological way a model of nursing which emphasises a physiological mode may not be for you. If your client has a disorder of mood rather than of body, a medical-adaptation approach may be of less relevance than one which has a bias towards psychological aspects of care. Most models combine all these but in differing degrees.

Still, you need not make use of any one model exclusively. In fact, it is wise not to, for the more models you consult the more ideas you have to hand. Often an eclectic approach works best where an individual's care takes the most appropriate parts of three or more models.

Personally I have found it useful to ask of each model three questions:

(1) How are clients perceived?
(2) What do nurses do?
(3) What is the nature of 'health' that nurses steer their clients towards?

The above questions provide a framework which enables me to understand how the subject model relates to those clients I have in mind, how similar my field view of nursing is to the model's perspective and if we share a like goal, namely, the same image of what contributes to health. I have chosen to discuss some of the more familiar models of care in the hope that this may help the reader to appreciate both the range and characteristics of these models. Use this information creatively and you may produce your own model. Models are not sacred; they are idea banks, resources to guide your own vision; so why not create your own model? Figure 1.4 may be of use in this; the earlier questions have been asked and a rough guide produced.

Fig. 1.4 A brief guide to the potential use of nursing models

Model	View of patient/client	What nurses do	Nature of health
Peplau	A unique system of biophysical and especially psychological traits and needs which interpersonally need direction	Facilitate renewed energy via the medium of the nurse–patient relationship	Optimum level of energy, when interpersonal and developmental activities are most productively performed
Henderson	Biological being with an interdependent relationship of body and mind	Help patients to meet 14 components of basic care related to: breathing, eating, eliminating waste, posture, sleep, dress, warmth, cleanliness, safety, communication, worship, work, play, learning	The ability for an individual to meet his own 14 components of care
Roy	Biological, psychological and sociological being who is attempting to adapt to an ever-changing environment. Further complicated by ill-health	Analyse problems and potential problems while working a process of assessment and problem-directed activity	One's position on a dynamic continuum of health–illness, ever subject to change
Orem	Individuals whose 'wholeness' has been fractured by illness and who need to realign their biological, sociological and symbolic function	Seek to overcome the limitations of illness via supporting the patient's ability for self-care	A condition of personal integrity where all parts work to complement a whole
King	Open systems with permeable boundaries which exchange physiological matter, emotional energy and social communication	Share a common situation where communication is mutually exchanged to set care objectives and work towards a common goal	Dynamic adjustment to internal and external stress so as to maximise living activity
Neuman	A physio-psycho-social being with cultural and developmental influences who needs help to maintain his wholeness via the dynamic balance of the above	Seek to reduce stresses of environment in order to re-establish totality of person	A constant state of flux depending upon the dynamic balance of the following four variables: physiologic, psychologic, sociocultural, developmental
Rogers	Four-dimensional energy field with unique pattern and organisation which show characteristic behaviours, not understandable by analysis of the parts	Seek to re-establish and promote interactive balance of environment and individual	Health is a value-laden word culturally denoting behaviours which are of high value

Fig. 1.4   (continued)

Model	View of patient/client	What nurses do	Nature of health
Fitzpatrick	Open system with continuous environmental interaction and characteristic life rhythms	Enhance development towards basic human rhythms and health	An ever-developing ability to encounter full potential and understand meaning of life

The worse thing that could happen would be for you to see only one model as providing the answer, following its script tightly and defending its rationale of care: better having no model than to worship one to the detriment of your own wider awareness. Models of care are not the answer, only one more step upon the way.

Postscript

It is both healthy and desirable that a wide range of nursing models exists along with the multitude of ideas, interpretations and conceptualisations of care they stimulate.

Nurses need to recognise the dichotomy that may arise between 'what they believe they do' and 'what the consequences of their actions actually are'. Nurses can humanise the formal demands of institutionalised care, serve as advocates on the client's behalf and offer counsel during times of trouble; they may likewise do the reverse of these things.

Nursing activity is diverse in the extreme; some nurses administer clinical care based on medical principles, others facilitate social learning, some work in the community, still others teach or administrate their fellows. Such behaviour makes it confusing, if not nigh impossible to develop one unifying professional model. Nurses employ applied knowledge and practise caring interventions. They may work from a 'scientific knowledge base' but 'caring is also an art'. No one philosophy, nor even a 'scientific' or 'applied art' perspective can fully justify all that nurses do.

It is from the diversity of a profession that its development occurs. Reduce these contrasts and you rob the profession of its growing edge. If we concur with the idea that nurses should be prepared to tolerate a multiplicity of care models in the clinical area and stay alive to the needs of those individuals they serve, we must likewise expect the profession itself to tolerate—and indeed welcome—a similar diversity in the body of its theory, values, beliefs, conceptualisations and practice. Having one main model may give an appearance of clarity, but it may also deny awareness of other perspectives. If nursing ever locates an all-inclusive model, in a similar way that physicians have done with medicine, then sadly it will also inherit those self-same faults it allocates to the medical profession.

If we really achieve clarity we may have to pay for it in terms of our personal sensitivity and professional tolerance; and once we have it what can we do with such clarity—force it upon others as the 'one and only way'? Better we remain attuned to the process of enquiry.

Critique

The way educationalists view nursing models differs significantly from that of nursing practitioners. The author in this chapter has conceptualised the salient points of a nursing-process approach, but as an educator emphasises conceptual awareness, personal sensitivity and the educative function models of nursing may have. Though a philosophical perspective is applied and the works of Menzies, Rogers and Heron are co-ordinated to a facilitation rôle framed by nursing rationale, perhaps more is made of nursing models than is useful. Perhaps the complexity of a multi-dimensional examination overshadows or even interferes with the practicalities of actually using models of care? If the previous argument is valid, the author could better have employed his time simplifying models of nursing rather than building further upon them.

A critique often made of the 1982 Syllabus of Training for the Mental Handicap Register is that it attempted to introduce subjects such as self-awareness without first preparing educators in techniques enabling the teaching of these; similarly, any change prescribed in nursing practice is doomed to fail unless it reaches the attitudinal base of the practitioner: as the author recognises such points in relation to the nursing process and seeks to prepare a foundation from which it can grow, possibly his approach is vindicated.

Paul Barber

Salient questions

1. Is the facilitator rôle described applicable to the nursing process?
2. Can the 'process' in nursing process be reduced to a social one?
3. Is the philosophy described applicable to clinical practice?
4. What constitutes the 'science' of nursing, and which elements or skills comprise its 'art'?
5. Is the above division of nursing into 'art' and 'science' a logical or meaningful one to make?
6. Is the nursing process the right and proper vehicle to correct the faults of the profession identified by the author?

References

Barber P 1986 The psychiatric nurse's failure therapeutically to nurture, *Nursing Practice*, No. 3, Longman Group, Harlow.

Bion WR 1961 *Experience in Groups*, Tavistock Publications, London.

Fitzpatrick JJ 1980 Patients' perceptions of time: current research, *Nursing Review*, **27**, 148–153.

Fitzpatrick JJ & Whall, AL 1983 *Conceptual Models of Nursing: Analysis and Application*, Prentice-Hall International.

Heron J 1975 *Six Category Intervention Analysis*, Human Potential Research Project, Department of Adult Education, University of Surrey.

Kilty J 1982 *Experiential Learning*, Human Potential Research Project, Department of Adult Education, University of Surrey.

Menzies I 1960 *The Functioning of Social Systems as a Defence Against Anxiety*, Tavistock Publications, London.

Orlando I 1961 *The Dynamic Nurse–Patient Relationship*, Putnam & Sons, New York.

Parse RS 1981 *Man–Living–Health: A Theory of Nursing*, John Wiley & Sons, New York.

Peplau HE 1952 *Interpersonal Relations in Nursing*, Putnam & Sons, New York.

Peplau HE 1968 Psychotherapeutic strategies, *Perspectives in Psychiatric Care*, **6**, 264–278.

Rogers C 1983 *Freedom to Learn in the Eighties*, Columbus.

Rogers M 1970 *An Introduction to the Theoretical Basis of Nursing*, F.A. Davies Co., Philadelphia.

Roy C 1979 Relating nursing theory to education: a new era, *Nurse Educator*, (March/April), 16–21.

World Health Organization 1976 *The Nursing Process*, WHO Document 06/08/77.

2

Putting community care together: a rationale for nursing interventions using Henderson's model of care—a community perspective

Amanda Gunner

Summary

This chapter documents those many reports which have combined to influence the care of mentally handicapped people. Here, the 'rôle' of the nurse is examined in the light of these sources, and advocacy is further linked to nursing action. Nurses as advocates of patient rights must of necessity be self-aware, and the experiential bias of the ENB Syllabus (1982) is viewed as attempting to address this. Similarly, the use of nursing models, which combine with earlier influence to emphasise the importance of 'person valuing' is seen to complement all that has gone before, providing a means whereby 'normalisation' may be implemented.

Maslow's hierarchy of human needs is introduced to clarify the range and character of need-related states. This needs-driven approach is incorporated to a needs-related model of nursing, namely, the vision of Virginia Henderson.

The care example of this chapter concerns itself with a client who is community-based, at home with her mother. Henderson's (1969) model is related to the assessment and planning of care goals as perceived by the Community Mental Handicap Team. Initial assessment is framed by Maslow's (1970) needs hierarchy, and subsequent identification of short- and long-term goals are individualised after Henderson and committed to care plan.

Paul Barber

Introduction

The last twenty years have seen enormous change enacted within the sphere of mental handicap. Persons suffering from this condition have moved from out of the shadow of institutional care and custodial systems of management to individualised modes within the community. Although this last area is in its infancy it has all the signs of being here to stay.

All this has come about due to a multitude of reasons, many linked to nurse training. Recently there has been a revised syllabus strongly invested with psycho-social skill training—*ENB (1982)*, a document that supports the use of nursing models and emphasises the rôle of the nurse as an educational force. This change occurred largely because of the following:

1. The RNMS training syllabus had failed to keep abreast with the times, being only superficially rearranged in 1970 to include sociology as a subject but no new skills.
2. The *Briggs Report (1972)* had called for complete educational revision.
3. The *Jay Report (1979)* and the *National Development Group Report* (1976–1980) had argued for a social context of care.
4. The Warnock Committee (1978) recommended the integration of handicapped children into mainstream education.
5. The East Nebraska Community Office of Retardation (1982) was widely reported in the

UK on its successful de-institutionalisation programme, and its message combined with the pressure of such groups as Royal Society for Mentally Handicapped Children & Adults (MENCAP), National Association for Mental Health (MIND), Campaign for Mental Handicap (CMH) and the Spastics Society who all advocated change on behalf of mentally handicapped people.

Sadly, from the above, it appears that nurses required the help of others to put their house in order.

The Preface of the new syllabus (*ENB*, 1982) states a philosophy which is based upon principles adopted by the United Nations in the Declaration of Human Rights (UN, 1978). It further states that the syllabus will prepare the student nurse to work within this philosophy and follow the rôle of the nurse as defined by Henderson (1969) using the skills of 'assessment, planning, implementation and evaluation based upon an identified body of knowledge' (*ENB*, 1982).

Awareness among nurses, other official bodies and the general public that mentally handicapped people have the same rights as everyone else further stimulated the move from an institutional mode to one of community care. However, it was generally recognised that a small proportion of profoundly multiply handicapped people will require full-time nursing care (Jay, 1979); too often this feature is conveniently forgotten. Those who support community care highlight the restrictive environment of the hospital setting and the over-protective and negative practices of the staff as reasons for the shift, and cite the work of Goffman (1961) in his ethnographic studies of 1954–1957. Because of this, many hospitals are fully aware of their short-comings and now seek to put them right; but a similar recognition of community 'problems' has yet to occur.

If integration is seen as becoming 'part of society', then the most applicable model of care for mentally handicapped people should logically be one that is socially aware. The concept of a social model of care has gradually replaced that of

the institution over the last 30 years, gaining most of its momentum over the last decade as the aforementioned reports—Jay (1979), National Development Group; the Briggs Report (1972)—percolated through a society awakened to civil rights and a nursing profession aware of the need to humanise its existent patterns of care.

These influences have stimulated the emergence of care provision based upon systematic nursing approaches which are now collectively seen as the '**nursing process**'. This term can best be seen as describing those 'cognitive', 'affective' and 'psychomotor activities' which determine the nurse's responses to individuals towards whom care is being directed. It is a framework for the organisation of nursing, not an encroachment upon the medical or para-medical professions. The nursing process facilitates individual understanding, aids recognition of those planning options available and assesses dynamically the interpersonal skill that may be enhanced to improve the quality of a client's life. Social awareness permeates this approach.

With increased social awareness, new rôles emerge such as advocacy. When nurses appreciate the socio-political constraints on care and feel strongly about their client's rights it is natural for them to fight for the relevant resources for such rights to be recognised and upheld; indeed, it becomes unethical not to do so. This aspect of the nursing process is considered unacceptable by some nurses, but it cannot be disregarded if nursing is to evolve the status of a right-acting committed client-centred profession.

Accountability should not merely be to senior management—a traditional feature of nursing—but to the patient; we are there to meet our patients' needs and voice their wants, and the greater their handicap, the greater their need for an advocate. The rôle of the nurse is thus essentially one of advocacy but, if nurses are to become effective advocates, assertion and self-awareness also become vital prerequisites (Code of Professional Conduct, UKCC, 1984). It is only through nurses' development of self-reflection upon their own feelings, thoughts, positive and negative communication that they will be able to generate effective care. Awareness training solicits a clearer understanding of just where our personal difficulties exist—especially those between us and the people for whom we care; such awareness may also suggest how we can go about trying to improve our interventions. If as nurses we wish to give those for whom we care a choice, then we must also develop 'our' insight and knowledge to choose. Without such training, nurses will suffer from a lack of professional vision, and there is an abundance of that around already.

Self-awareness can also be developed through introspection, where the outcomes of past and present approaches to 'clinical problem-solving' are evaluated, but for this to happen we need to appreciate how 'past' systems of care differ from the 'present' ones we employ; records are therefore essential.

Figure 2.1 suggests a strategy and formalises one such route of problem identification worthy of recording: the solid arrows show a cyclical process; if you attempt this route and having worked though the cycle find a solution is still not forthcoming, the broken line indicates a path where re-assessment and modification coexist and can continue to clarify the issues addressed. This sort of problem-solving framework underpins much of the nursing process, and although simplistic initiates a reflective exercise from whence personal awareness may spring.

Self-awareness may similarly be developed through experience—something of which all nurses have a wealth—but they must have the opportunity to reflect on their own exploratory processes, share these with their peers, and discuss those alternatives which open out before them. Doing a task without self-awareness is useless here. The self-disclosure and empathy that may develop between nurses from such experiential sharing may be similarly enacted in the nurse–client relationship; indeed, the concept of 'learning from experience' is central to the

Fig. 2.1   Process of problem identification and solving

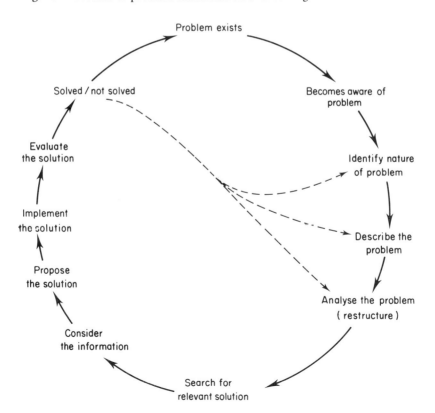

1982 Syllabus and the rising use of experiential teaching methods. But caution here—it is wise to remember that self-awareness is but one part of effective nursing and must be synonymous with knowledge. Knowledge orientates, experiential awareness provides an appreciation of 'reality', and reflection enriches self-understanding. Nursing models encourage this link; they conceptualise care, suggest interventions, generate further knowledge by the enquiries they make and encourage personal and professional reflection.

A philosophical base for care

The view inherent in all nursing models is that each person is a unique individual to be valued, regardless of their skill level, intellect, status position or health. In trying to evolve a model of care, one must be cautious; it would be all too easy to fall into the trap of using a model of care and fitting the individual into it. This is temptingly easy to fall into when your clients are non-assertive, slow of response or impoverished in ideas. Not involving the family in the care process can be one more means of devaluing the resident.

To be able to state that 'anyone who cares for people who are mentally handicapped never devalues them in any way' is an absolute statement, and though ideal is scarcely ever achieved.

At one level, the act of isolating them in hospital, hostel, or other specialist caring institution undermines their social status; at a personal level we may individually fear, patronise or treat them as eternal children.

Principles must be based on theories, be they biological, sociological, psychological or humanistic. The knowledge base must grow from clinical reality and perform a critical evaluation of the living and learning environment in total. A starting point might well arise from an adaptation of Maslow's hierarchy model of human needs (Figure 2.2). An example of how this may be employed in evaluation of a client's initial care needs will be provided in the subsequent care example.

If one looks at McFarlane and Castledine's (1982) 'summary of statements about the nature of nursing', two stand out as especially interrelated to our discussion so far:

1. Nursing has to do with meeting basic human needs for life and health.
2. Nursing has to do with meeting the deficiencies of people in carrying out daily living activities, i.e. with deficits in self-care ability.

Physiological needs and bodily maintenance via medical intervention and the provision of safety are easily achieved, but what of helping another to reach full potential and feel actualised—how do you plan for this in care? Maslow's need

Fig. 2.2   Maslow's hierarchy of human needs (after Maslow, 1970)

Health orientations	Care requirements
Best/most fulfilling experiences	Self-actualisation needs
Beauty/order/understanding	Aesthetic needs
Educational fulfillment	Cognitive needs
Status/respect for self	Esteem needs
Social acceptance/feedback	Belongingness and love needs
Environmental security	Safety needs
Bodily maintenance/health	Physiological needs

model is therefore useful in orientating us conceptually to the broad bands of interest which compile the care spectrum. It does not provide answers—that's our job—it just sharpens up our perception and helps us step outside the traditional perspective we all too often share.

The basis of normalisation, a concept which accords with this view, is, according to Nirje (1976), that 'A person is a person first, the handicap is secondary'. Each person has the right to live, interact and develop in a healthy and positive environment. Within this will be reflected values, ideas and attitudes as the individual adapts to this environment and it in turn responds to him.

The concept of normalisation, although apparently simple, has far-reaching implications for all aspects of care provision offered to mentally handicapped people. It seeks to stimulate the acceptance of persons (handicapped) within 'normal' society. Normalisation does not equate with normality, a popular misconception. If nurses are to enhance and preserve the human dignity of their clients, they will have to share their professional power base more and avoid the trap of 'devaluing responses to people with mental handicap' (Tyne, 1978). Devaluing responses are common to handicap care, and seem to arise naturally as an 'us and them' mentality:

(a) *Dehumanisation*—treating people with mental handicap as if they are less worthy than others who are normal and gainfully employed.
(b) *Age appropriateness*—treating people with mental handicaps as if they are—and always will be—children. The nurse as parent who always decides for them and acts on their behalf.
(c) *Isolation*—segregating people with mental handicaps away from valued communities and valued people, the historical legacy of hospitalised care.

Exercises

1. Consider how you, as a nurse could help to avoid the above devaluing responses in your clinical area. How might you prepare junior staff to reverse the effects of isolation for your clients? Try and list ways of preventing the above.

Nurses cannot work in a vacuum, but if care is given based on rituals, albeit unconscious, then as specialists providing specialist care we will rapidly become extinct. The rôle of the nurse must surely be based upon updated knowledge. For many, this devaluing process reveals itself in the form of language used when relating to people who are mentally handicapped, i.e. pet names, child-like terms and the use of over-familiarity.

2. Mentally list all the words that you have used or heard others use to describe someone who is mentally handicapped. Now, reflect upon your list. What is your immediate reaction? Do some of the words or phrases make you cringe, laugh or perhaps even evoke no reaction?

Awareness of how the carer herself feels affects both the care and the way in which it is given. The definition in the 1982 Syllabus (adapted from Henderson, 1969) states:

> The function of the nurse for people with mental handicap is directly and skillfully to assist the individual and his family, whatever the handicap, in the acquisition, development and maintenance of those skills that, given the necessary ability—and preparation—could be performed unaided; and to do this in such a way as to enable independence to be gained as rapidly and fully as possible, in an environment that maintains a quality of life that would be acceptable to fellow citizens of the same age.

Henderson sees basic nursing care as applicable to any setting, home, school or workplace, and states:

> that the better the example the nurse sets the more likely she is to influence others constructively.

Here we may appreciate the nurse's social educational rôle. The following list consists of 'The components of basic nursing care' as set down by Henderson (1969).

1. Helping patient with respiration.
2. Helping patient with eating and drinking.
3. Helping patient with elimination.
4. Helping patient maintain desirable posture in walking, sitting, and lying; and helping him with moving from one position to another.
5. Helping patient rest and sleep.
6. Helping patient with selection of clothing, with dressing and undressing.
7. Helping patient maintain body temperature within normal range.
8. Helping patient keep body clean and well groomed and protect integument.
9. Helping patient avoid dangers in the environment; and protecting others from any potential dangers from the patient, such as infection or violence.
10. Helping patient communicate with others—to express his needs and feelings.
11. Helping patient practise his religion or conform to his concept of right or wrong.
12. Helping patient with work, or productive occupation.
13. Helping patient with recreational activities.
14. Helping patient learn.

A community experience

> The Community Mental Handicap Team (CMHT) is not intended to be a substitute for any existing service, nor is it intended to cover all mentally handicapped children and adults.
> (Simon, 1981)

In keeping with the above quote, the CMHT await referrals before acting. The weekly meeting of the team makes sure that impending and new cases are brought to everyone's attention as soon as possible. This gives an opportunity for discussion and the planning of the initial home visit and preliminary assessment, which is usually carried out by one or two members of the CMHT, the core of which are the specialist nurse and social worker; extra support comes from psychologists and doctors as requested.

The first home visit gives the chance to obtain not only a degree of assessment, but an accurate case history—if this is not already available. Further assessment, if necessary, may be carried out by other team members at school, the adult training centre or the client's home. Once the initial assessment is completed and recommendations have been made, a key worker will be appointed to ensure implementation of actions and to maintain contact with the family.

Sharon and Mrs Green—a care example

In the following care example I will attempt to show how concepts of normalisation, social awareness and the use of the Henderson model of nursing may be combined to care for a severely mentally handicapped girl living with her mother in the community. There will perhaps be times when I fail to achieve my own ideals; if so, contemplate how else care may have been conveyed.

In this particular instance, Sharon and her mother, Mrs Green, were referred to the CMHT by a member of their community, the local vicar. The problem—as seen by the vicar—was one of support for the family, especially Mrs Green, particularly as Sharon, now 26 years old and severely mentally handicapped, had never been apart from her mother. Mrs Green had on many occasions confided in the vicar her anxiety of not being able to cope with her daughter's daily care.

The weekly team meeting brought forward several points for discussion on the scant information available:

1. Gain a more detailed history relating to Sharon and her mother in an attempt to establish the nature of the situation and any problems which may exist.
2. Find out from Mrs Green what she would like to see achieved in terms of future or expected success.
3. Establish with Mrs Green and Sharon what was acceptable in tackling any needs or problems, i.e. methods and agencies that may be used.

4. Find out whether Mrs Green felt she wanted any help and if the CMHT were the most appropriate agency

It was suggested that the nurse for that particular portion of the catchment area where the family lived would be accompanied by the vicar on her first visit. This was arranged for the middle of that same week.

At this point, it is appropriate to remember that both Sharon and her mother were considered priorities. To involve the family is essential, but the point is often missed by professionals that every mentally handicapped person has—or has had—parents. This may seem obvious, but for community-based professionals the authority of the family is often seen as in competition with their own—so they ignore it. This separation of the client's problem from their parents' will often not be an intentional act.

> But if we recognise this can happen, it may be the beginning of a better understanding of the problems of the mentally handicapped child and his family.
>
> (Hannam, 1983)

Bearing this in mind, the following extract summarises the relevant information gained by the community nurse during the first few visits to the Green family, and her sensitivity to the family unit.

Visits to the Green family

Initial visit
The community nurse duly accompanied the vicar on the first visit to the Green family. Mrs Green seemed somewhat alarmed by the presence of the nurse and consequently carried out her conversation to both the vicar and nurse from the front door and did not offer an opportunity for either party to enter the house. Every so often Mrs Green would shout at Sharon to be quiet but neither the vicar nor nurse saw Sharon—although she could be heard screaming at regular intervals.

When the nurse asked Mrs Green if she would like her to visit again, next week, Mrs Green accepted readily and stated that the same day and time would be most convenient.

The initial visit seemed to achieve little in establishing any real information regarding those problems Mrs Green and her daughter might be experiencing. The vicar had previously stated that Mrs Green was particularly suspicious of the 'welfare people', and that to his knowledge, only he and one other neighbour ever entered the house. Information at this stage was very brief, but sufficient for speculation on what the initial assessment needed to address and the questions to be asked.

The following team meeting suggested that weekly visits should continue. Maslow's need model was consulted (see Figure 2.3). This served to focus team attention and awareness upon those options available and the probable interventions required.

Subsequent visits
Weekly visits over the following month were carried out on the doorstep of the house and the needs of the family further investigated. A little more information was gained each time, although Sharon was never seen, only heard. The initial orientation of Maslow's hierarchy was tempered by reality. It was established that Mrs Green was in her late seventies and had been married and widowed three times.

Sharon was the only child of her second marriage, and although a married daughter from Mrs Green's first marriage was a frequent visitor to the house and heavily relied upon by her mother, it was felt unwise to depend too much on her on-going support as she lived some fifty miles away. Alternative support was therefore necessary.

On the fifth visit, the community nurse was invited into the house and met Sharon for the first time. Talking to Mrs Green over a cup of tea—while observing the interaction of Sharon and her mother—became the nature of the weekly visit. The house was very old and damp and lacking a bathroom. A toilet had been built on to the kitchen but was too narrow for Mrs Green to see to Sharon, and so a commode kept in the back-room was used instead.

Fig. 2.3 Initial assessment brief based on Maslow's need model

Assessment focus	Family/client needs suggested	Nursing options available
Physiological needs	To prevent Mrs Green becoming over-exhausted. Help Sharon to function independently	Teach Sharon more self-maintenance skills; bathing, skin-care, general grooming. Help Mrs Green appreciate the need for Sharon to do more for herself
Safety needs	For Sharon to appreciate the dangers of her environment	Teach Sharon a little more 'road-sense' so that she may understand her mother's intentions more when they are out together
Belonging needs	Sharon's present social isolation and her mother's need for a break from twenty-four hour care needs to be considered	Introduce Sharon and her mother to local community support groups, clubs and parents' groups
Esteem needs	For Sharon to have an area of function where she may feel special	Assess Sharon's hobbies, skills, or ability to perform jobs she gets satisfaction from around the home
Cognitive needs	For Sharon to reach her social and intellectual potential	Assess Sharon's baseline skill levels and introduce family to agencies who may develop these skills
Aesthetic needs	For family to understand the rationale behind the suggestions for care, to contribute to the logic of these and work together with care staff towards shared goals	Let Mrs Green and Sharon list those needs/aims they see as important and suggest activities to meet these; produce shared short-term goals for all to measure care by
Self-actualisation	For Sharon and her mother to maximise their enjoyment and fulfilment, and to appreciate life together	Find out family's most treasured activities, give encouragement and opportunity for these, especially where joint ventures occur.

Sharon seemed to spend all her time on the move, stamping her way through the lower rooms of the house and screaming. Sharon was a tall, well-built young lady given to bouts of self-mutilation, when she would pinch, prick or bang herself, causing numerous bruises and cuts. Mrs Green said that when Sharon's mutilation became 'very bad' she would give her tablets (Largactil, 100 mg) but, she also said that she did not like giving the tablets and would sometimes not bother. The initial assessment brief (Figure 2.3) had correctly appreciated the physiological and belonging needs of the family.

Mrs Green's main concern over Sharon's health was her eating. She felt very strongly that Sharon's problem of hyperactivity and mutilation could be helped by feeding her puréed food at regular set times. Goal-setting was necessary, and Henderson's model was employed as a nursing aid to focus upon the major problem areas. Figure 2.4 shows the outcome. The awarenesses that arose from this were then put to the test—and evaluated within the context of later visits.

Over the next three visits, the community nurse tried to establish Mrs Green's feelings

Fig. 2.4   Identification of possible short-term goals based on Henderson's model

Helping	Short-term goals	Long-term goals
With respiration	Assess possible needs here	
With eating/drinking	Show Mrs Green ways of developing Sharon's self-feeding	Self-feeding by Sharon and a more normal diet, non-purée
With elimination	Educate Mrs Green to the management of a more balanced diet for Sharon	Roughage, fruit as part of diet; grant to enlarge toileting area
Maintain desirable posture	Assess possible needs here	
Rest/sleep	To gain more rest for Mrs Green; 8 hours' sleep to be achieved per night	Holidays with support for the family via appropriate agencies
Select clothing/ dress–undress	Encourage Mrs Green to allow Sharon more say in her dress	Sharon to be taken shopping for her own clothes and involved in the selection
Maintain body temperature	Assess possible needs here	
Keep clean/groomed	Sharon to be trained in self-grooming skills	Sharon to wash and groom herself with the minimum of supervision by her mother
Avoid danger/protect others	For Mrs Green to record those events causing self-mutilation	For Mrs Green to understand when Sharon may self-mutilate and identify preventative measures
Communicate needs/ feelings	Help Mrs Green to feel less isolated and more supported in her care of Sharon	
Practise religion/conform to her beliefs of right/wrong	Assess possible needs here	
With work	Encourage Sharon to extend her hours at the ATC and for Mrs Green to be enabled to perform her housework without interruption	For Sharon and her mother to share in home maintenance
With recreational activities	Enrich Mrs Green's activity range to overcome her feelings of being trapped	For Sharon and her mother to share a holiday together with support
Learn	To introduce the family to others within the community who they may share with, and gain support from, plus psychologist	For Sharon to understand her own needs and begin to appreciate herself and others more, and gain toileting skills

about the future. The nurse gave Mrs Green information about the sources and agencies that could help and exactly what they were offering, addressing especially Mrs Green's 'feelings' regarding her isolation from supportive agencies and releasing her dependence on her eldest daughter.

The one agency that seemed to interest Mrs Green was the local Adult Training Centre, mainly it seemed, because it was only two miles away! The nurse suggested that if Mrs Green would like to visit the Centre this could be arranged, but that the manager of the Adult Training Centre would also like to meet Sharon. The Adult Training Centre was felt to be both a potential area for Sharon to gain 'productive occupation' and 'self-esteem', and for her mother to gain a rest from continual care demands.

The visit to the Adult Training Centre took place two weeks later but was not without its problems. On arriving to pick up Mrs Green and Sharon—in order to take them to the Centre—Mrs Green seemed very anxious and expressed this by saying she was sure that Sharon would not be able to travel in the car as she was not used to travelling in any form of transport. After this comment, the short journey was apprehensive from everyone's point of view! However, there were no problems and the visit to the Centre went well. The manager stated that a place was available for Sharon, beginning with a half-day a week on Wednesdays. Mrs Green said she would think about the proposal.

The identification process (shown in Figure 2.4) motivated further care planning. At this point, the reader should refer to the ongoing care plan devised by the community nurse based on Henderson's model. This served as the daily work plan and superseded the earlier initial assessment and reflected the goal-planning. It should be noted that the front sheet—containing referral, personal, and history details—is not included, and that review is scheduled on a weekly basis (Figure 2.5).

The care plan includes an example of four of the possible fourteen components of Henderson's basic nursing care. The goals are a mixture of short, medium and long term. This is important, as too many long-term goals tend to hinder progress, the target seeming to be unattainable. Nurses kept one eye on the initial assessment sheet (Figure 2.3), and another on the problem identification chart (Figure 2.4) when developing subsequent care strategies. The 'ongoing care plan' fed reality back to earlier conceptions the care team had made. This is not to say it was definitive; it too was under constant revision. Planning of new care and continuing evaluation is therefore seen as a never-ceasing process. The care plan thus serves as a record of the story so far, those insights that arose, and a progress marker of the direction of care. As one care goal is reached, further goals are suggested.

Continuation of the care study
The following two months brought progress. After five weeks of attending the ATC for half a day everyone agreed that Sharon should spend all of Wednesday there. Within a month of this progress her attendance was again increased to one-and-a-half days a week. And within another month, Sharon's attendance increased to two days a week—Wednesday and Friday.

Exercises

1. Living with uncertainty is essential in nursing. The reader is invited to enter further future possible goals—bearing in mind the information so far—and to enlarge upon the care and modify what has gone before. For instance, what short- and long-term goals might be suggested to acclimatise Sharon to travelling?
2. How could you improve upon the mode of care described?

Conclusion

This chapter has explored the use of a model of nursing in caring for people who are mentally handicapped. It has done so with one model in particular—the Henderson (1961) basic principles of care—and has complemented this

Fig. 2.5   Care plan

Helping the client/family with:	Goal (long–medium–short)	Nursing care	Suggestions for those giving care
Communication with others and to express her needs and feelings	Mrs Green will feel able to contact the CMHT herself, when she feels Sharon or she herself needs help (*long term*)	To visit the home once a week and actively listen to Mrs Green	If asked by Mrs Green how to deal with a given need, then offer advice and leave her to make the decision. Possibility of involving the Good Neighbour Scheme
Work/production	Mrs Green will be able to shop and carry out her housework twice weekly, without having to leave Sharon with her neighbour (*long term*)	To escort Sharon to and from the ATC on Wednesday afternoons, until corporation transport can be arranged. Assess Sharon's ability to perform simple household chores	Pick up Sharon at 13.30 hours. Return her home at 16.00 hours. Ask the ATC to write a diary that will also be kept by Mrs Green. It will be the communication between them regarding Sharon.
Recreational activities	Mrs Green will have a regular activity which is outside her home, mixing with her own peer group (*medium term*)	Offer alternatives of activities Mrs Green could do when Sharon is at the ATC	Take brochures and literature on activities that seem to interest Mrs Green, e.g. club and social meetings connected with church and local area. Holidays for parents with handicapped children
	To organise an annual holiday for Sharon and her mother (*short term*)	Contact the local Mencap branch regarding holidays	Find out details of places, accommodation and costs
	Sharon will spend five minutes a day throwing ball to: her mother, a member of the ATC staff (named), and the community nurse (*medium term*)	Liaise with the ATC and the psychologist to draw up a programme	Involve Mrs Green in planning and implementing the programme. Buy a ball!
Learning	Sharon will be able to pull up her pants after she has used the toilet (*short term*)	Liaise with the ATC and the psychologist to draw up a programme	Involve Mrs Green in planning and implementing the programme. Mrs Green and the community nurse to carry out the programme at the ATC then to try at home

approach by reference to 'normalisation' and Maslow's hierarchy of human needs. Although it is very tempting to fit the individual to 'the model', what has been attempted is rather the adaptation of a specific model which

> is applicable to the care of any patient . . . . . but which does not 'describe method' and is 'in no sense a manual'.
>
> (Henderson, 1969)

A flexible approach has therefore been suggested. It is up to the nurse to take the 'basic principles of care' and use these relevantly for their client's welfare, so enabling the planning, implementing and evaluating of individualised care, once they have ascertained the particular merits and needs of their client's unique situation. Figure 2.6 encapsulates this process, relating it to the community example of this chapter, the inter-relationship of the initial assessment, 'formulation of goals', and 'ongoing care plan'. In looking at the word 'model', one could view it from the definition appropriate to the following analogy: in the fashion world the latest clothes

look great on a model—but it does not mean that they will suit you. The same view can be taken with regard to models of nursing care. They are something to look at, they give ideas but should not control the present situations or end result; they are growing points, tools of enquiry. We should never aim to make the model successful in itself, only relevant to the care at hand and complementary to the client's needs and the nurse's skill. Models of nursing are simply the media through which we may create and express our care.

Critique

One may speculate that the rôle of the community nurse is primarily a socially orientated one, and as such would be better served by a social adaptation model of care. Why then use Henderson, whose tabulation of human needs seems overweighted to a biological perspective? Is the aforementioned model therefore relevant to community care?

Though superficially Henderson's model appears

Fig. 2.6 Care stages in relationship to the problem-solving process

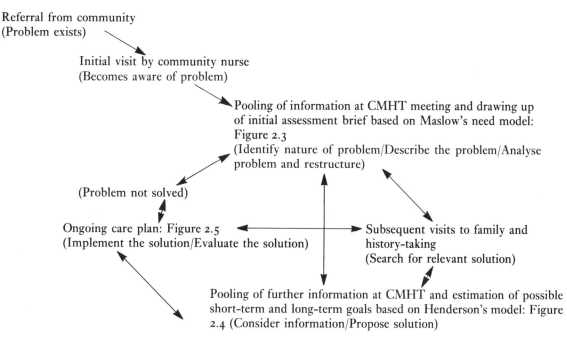

Referral from community
(Problem exists)

Initial visit by community nurse
(Becomes aware of problem)

Pooling of information at CMHT meeting and drawing up of initial assessment brief based on Maslow's need model: Figure 2.3
(Identify nature of problem/Describe the problem/Analyse problem and restructure)

(Problem not solved)

Ongoing care plan: Figure 2.5
(Implement the solution/Evaluate the solution)

Subsequent visits to family and history-taking
(Search for relevant solution)

Pooling of further information at CMHT and estimation of possible short-term and long-term goals based on Henderson's model: Figure 2.4 (Consider information/Propose solution)

little related to the community, when we examine more closely her approach, certain assumptions are revealed to underline her work.

1. Independence is the key objective towards which client and nurse direct their activity.
2. The concept of health is a socially derived one equated with independence.
3. Nurses facilitate patients to health while appreciating them as 'integrated wholes'.
4. Though a limited number of needs exist, there is an infinite number of ways to meet these needs.

In retrospect, the above seem to do nothing to detract from socially dynamic practice; the author seems fittingly to have employed the above qualities, but would an alternative model have been more appropriate? As the scale of care was directed towards the family unit, possibly the principles of care suggested by Henderson were more appropriate than other more individualised models that focus upon specifics rather than general themes.

Paul Barber

Salient questions

1. What other model might have been appropriate to community nursing care?
2. What factors may interfere with the concept of the nurse as an advocate of patient rights?
3. How could the client have been more involved in the planning of her own care goals?
4. Was the care described predominantly client-centred or nurse-derived?

References

Department of Education and Science 1978 *Special Educational Needs, The Warnock Report.* HMSO, London.

Department of Health and Social Security 1971 *Better Services for the Mentally Handicapped.* HMSO, London.

DRG 1977 *Mentally Handicapped Children: A Plan for Action 2.* DHSS, London.

DRG 1977 *Helping Mentally Handicapped School Leavers 3.* DHSS, London.

English National Board 1982 *Syllabus of Training Professional Register, Part 5.* ENB, London.

Goffman E 1961 *Asylums: Essays on the Social Situation of Mental Patients and Other Inmates.* Penguin, London.

Hannam C 1983 Bringing up a mentally handicapped child: the parents' point of view. In: Tierney A (ed) *Nurses and the Mentally Handicapped.* John Wiley, Chichester.

Henderson V 1969 *Basic Principles of Nursing Care* (revised edition). S. Karger, Basel and New York.

Hewitt JP 1941 *Self and Dosiceyt: A Symbolic Interactionist Social Psychology.* 3rd edition. Allyn & Bacon Inc, Newton MA, USA.

Jay Committee 1979 *Report of the Committee into Mental Handicapped Nursing Care.* DHSS, London.

McFarlane J & Castledine G 1982 *A Guide to the Practice of Nursing Using the Nursing Process.* CV Mosby Co., St Louis.

Maslow AH 1970 *Motivation and Personality.* 2nd edition. Harper & Row, New York.

Mental Health Act 1959. HMSO, London.

National Development Group 1976 *Mental Handicap—Planning Together—1.* DHSS, London.

Nirje B 1976 The normalisation principle. In: Kugel R & Shearer A (eds) *Changing Patterns of Residential Services for the Mentally Retarded.* Presidents Committee for the Mentally Retarded.

Simon GB 1981 *Local Services for the Mentally Handicapped.* British Institute of Mental Handicap.

Tyne 1978 *Looking at Life in a Hospital, Hostel, Home or Unit.* CMH.

3

Initiating the use of a nursing model: the importance of systematic care planning— a ward clinician's perspective

John Aldridge

Summary
This chapter examines the need for thorough nursing assessment and demonstrates the use which can be made of this when formulating care strategies. Normalisation is addressed, as is the nurse's rôle in promoting appropriate social behaviour. Care plans are many and diverse, and serve to narrate the direction that nursing interventions take, while describing the emergence of the rationale on which these are based. The frustrations that attend the 'management of change' are described and serve to warn us of those obstacles traditional practice poses to a nursing-model approach. Finally, the author re-evaluates his approach and suggests a new model more readily applicable to the care of mentally handicapped people.

Paul Barber

The context

This chapter describes the care of a severely handicapped young man using an appropriate model of nursing and concerns itself with the initiation of a care programme over some five weeks. The clinical culture for which the programme was intended was one unfamiliar with 'model-based' performance; it was therefore necessary to initiate change gradually, so that staff might orientate themselves more easily to the rationale and skills involved.

Although there were well-known models to choose from (Roper, 1980; Roy, 1970) none

seemed wholly suited to the care of mentally handicapped people. An eclectic approach was therefore employed which combined aspects of many models.

Aggleton and Chalmers (1984) observe that all nursing models must say something about:

1. The nature of the people receiving (or about to receive) nursing care.
2. Causes of problems that are likely to require nursing intervention.
3. The nature of the assessment process.
4. The nature of planning and goal-setting.
5. The focus of nursing intervention during implementation of a care plan.
6. The nature of the process of evaluating the quality and effects of the care provided.

None of the models familiar to me addressed the above in terms of mentally handicapped people. There was, for instance, an underlying emphasis on illness which runs contrary to contemporary care. Gunzburg (1973) states that

> Mental handicap is not a mental illness; it is mostly an unfortunate state to which one is born. . . . . .

He further declares that the concept of absolute illness, though not necessarily wrong, is misleading when applied to mental handicap because it diverts staff attention from social re-education and systematic assessment and thus overlooks a major tenet of handicap care, namely, that:

> The assessment of social competence in the sense of assessing skills of conforming provides a

systematic technique of exploring the ingredients which contribute towards social adjustment in the mentally handicapped and is thus an essential procedure for directing and planning his social education and training.

(Gunzburg, 1973)

In recent years literature has been published concerning the use of client-centred modes of care for mentally handicapped persons; such sources (Bowness and Zadik, 1981; Leslie and Shiells, 1981; Samy, 1983a and 1983b; Green, 1984) do not use the central concept of a social skills approach or overtly describe a model of nursing but they do provide a conceptual foundation on which to build.

Attention has been drawn, however, to methods of social evaluation which may be combined with these sources to effect person-centred assessments. Bailey (1982) suggests that there are in existence a number of assessment tools specially developed for use with mentally handicapped people. For instance, many nurses are already familiar with the use of Gunzburg's Progress Assessment Charts (PAC) and the Adaptive Behavior Scale (ABS) described by Nihira *et al.* (1974).

The PAC and ABS were seen to be appropriate to the care described in this chapter for the following reasons:

(a) Both tools were already in use within the client's clinical area.
(b) Both conformed with the recommendations of Gunzburg (1973) in that they systematically address social competence.
(c) Both tools were designed for use with a mentally handicapped population.

There is, however, no reason why other assessment tools should not be used as long as these are 'relevant' to your area.

The case of Geoff

The client's background

Before describing actual assessment and care, a short history and background of the client described in this text is necessary.

Geoff was born in August 1962 and at the time of this study was aged 23. In October 1965 he was diagnosed by a consultant paediatrician as autistic. Letters dated in 1965 state that he was able to vocalise and spoke one or two words; another of 1967 describes 'distractable and repetitive behaviour, and that he was routine-oriented and had special fears'. He was admitted to the local mental handicap hospital in 1972 and transferred to his present ward in 1980. A psychologist's assessment in 1983 estimated a mental age of 15 months and a social age of less than three years, and further observed that behaviour was stereotypic and ritualistic in character. As a consequence of this, Geoff showed a short attention span. A home visit by a community mental handicap nurse reported that when Geoff is at home (usually every weekend) his parents describe obsessional behaviour and that he is self-injurious (smacking his ears and occasionally head-banging) if his routine is upset or if he is thwarted. Therefore, they give in rather than risk upsetting him. A speech therapist's report of June 1985 stated that in symbolic play he was confined to real and large objects, appropriate to a developmental age of 12–13 months. In language it was thought that he could understand about six Amerind signs (this is the sign system in use in the hospital). He had no executive use of speech, but seemed to have good verbal understanding, though this was largely situational. Much use was made of body language and facial expression. Vocalisation would seem to have become extinct, possibly due to the absence of any environmental reinforcement.

At the time of my involvement, Geoff was, and had for some time been posing a number of problems to the ward. He was a very active young man and due to his size (6ft 1 in) and weight (15st 10 lb) was difficult to handle both on the ward and in the training department, which he attended each morning. He was however very likeable, though with very few social skills and with just sufficient self-help skills to make him relatively independent in a ward of severely handicapped men. His behaviour, though containing some features of autism, was in many ways similar to that of many other severely handi-capped people who have spent a number of years in institutional care. In addition to these insights my initial notes observed that he had few skills in self-amusement; this, combined with his often overactive behaviour and sheer size contributed to his labelling by staff as a 'problem' and led to his frequent exclusion from the training depart-ment at times of staff sickness and shortage. Geoff's parents, although still closely involved with him, had not developed nor been allowed to develop a close and 'honest' relationship with the ward that would have been therapeutic to them. Nursing interventions and family interventions therefore occurred in isolation from one another. There was no evidence that there had been any concerted nursing based on a rational identi-fication of Geoff's problems, i.e. no nursing aims were recorded; the situation was one that could best be described as a 'holding situation' and was far from ideal for Geoff, his parents or the ward.

The following practical and ethical consider-ations were kept in mind.

1. That Geoff had been a long-term resident in hospital and that I would be breaking into an already-established complex of relationships and would thus need tact and sensitivity to change these therapeutically in any way.
2. Any therapeutic work of the nature intended would, of necessity, be of a very tentative kind, and be directed to long-term results.
3. I had no ethical right to establish a re-lationship with the family that would not, or could not, be sustained once commenced.

It was noted that Geoff's parents should not be led into expectations that could not be realised, for this would cause unnecessary distress.

The assessment procedure

Before attempting any constructive nursing I spent one week in observation of Geoff in order to know him better. During this week I kept a diary of my own unstructured observations (which I maintained throughout the period of involvement) and completed the PAC and ABS assessment tools. I would suggest now that this may be too short a period in which to attempt a comprehensive assessment, but this insight developed from hindsight.

I now appreciate the view of Jean Crow (1979), who states that

If insufficient time or trouble is taken over assess-ment, fewer patient problems will be identified.

It is a valid and a valuable lesson to have learned. A nursing care plan can only be as good as the information on which it is based.

My initial observations of Geoff led me to choose the Gunzburg PAC as a starting point for assessment. This was completed by scoring according to the PAC Manual Vol. 1 which gives detailed criteria against which one may measure a client's performance (Gunzburg, 1977). I follo-wed the suggested method when filling in the wheel-like diagram by using dark shading for an item that has been satisfactorily completed, light shading for items that have been tested but not satisfactorily completed, and left blank those items that had not been tested.

Geoff scored well in the Self Help section, having scored on all but sections concerning drying hands and unbuttoning. The Occupation section was also completed with only a few 'fails'—though I bore in the back of my mind the difference between being able to do something and doing it regularly of one's own volition. In the areas of Communication and Socialisation however, Geoff scored very low and very patch-ily. Further assessment of this area was deemed desirable, as Geoff's main needs, and indeed the focus for subsequent nursing interventions, were primarily located in the domain of communi-cation and social behaviour.

A more 'socially specific' assessment tool was necessary for further investigation and clarific-ation of Geoff's abilities, and to this end the AAMD Adaptive Behavior Scale was filled, scored, and then interpreted according to the ABS manual. This is a lengthy assessment tool, but produces thorough social data for use in problem identification. Figure 3.1 demonstrates the nature of that data the Adaptive Behavior

Fig. 3.1   Data summary sheet 1

Identification	Geoff W.
Age	24
Sex	M
Date of Administration	3/2/84

DATA SUMMARY SHEET-AAMD ADAPTIVE BEHAVIOR SCALE PART ONE

A. Eating 11
B. Toilet Use 5
C. Cleanliness.................................... 7
D. Appearance 6
E. Care of Clothing 0
F. Dressing & Undressing 5
G. Travel................................ 1
H. General Independent Functioning 1

  I. INDEPENDENT FUNCTIONING ⟶ 36   I

A. Sensory Development 6
B. Motor Development.. 16

  II. PHYSICAL DEVELOPMENT ⟶ 22   II

A. Money Handling and Budgeting 0
B. Shopping Skills.................................... 0

  III. ECONOMIC ACTIVITY ⟶ 0   III

A. Expression 2
B. Comprehension........................... 0
C. Social Language Development...................... 0

  IV. LANGUAGE DEVELOPMENT ⟶ 2   IV

  V. NUMBERS AND TIME ⟶ 0   V

A. Cleaning 0
B. Kitchen Duties 0
C. Other Domestic Activites 0

  VI. DOMESTIC ACTIVITY ⟶ 0   VI

  VII. VOCATIONAL ACTIVITY ⟶ 0   VII

A. Initiative 0
B. Perseverance........................... 0
C. Leisure Time 0

  VIII. SELF-DIRECTION ⟶ 0   VIII

  IX. RESPONSIBILITY ⟶ 0   IX

  X. SOCIALIZATION ⟶ 0   X

Scale uncovers; the higher the numerical rating, the greater the degree of competency shown by a client. A data summary sheet, such as the one illustrated, provides a good guide for nursing action.

One of the reasons for which I decided to use the ABS was to compare its use to the PAC. It is interesting to note that both give similar results. Independent Functioning (or Self Help) and Physical Development are both scored high. The ABS taps areas in addition to the PAC, in that it assesses items of maladaptive behaviour. This could be seen as a rather negative way of looking at mentally handicapped people but it does have the advantage of allowing one to compare a client's strengths and weaknesses, both 'practical' and 'behavioural'.

Provided one retains a balanced view, looking at both positive and negative aspects, it results in a more complete evaluation; as Figure 3.2 demonstrates.

The raw scores given in the data summary sheets do not have much meaning in themselves—it is necessary to convert these scores to a more meaningful graph form by reference to standardised tables in the ABS manual. These tables allow one to compare the scores attained by one's client with scores attained by other mentally handicapped people of the same sex and similar age range; it is here that one begins to find interesting results.

The ABS divides its Profile Summary into two parts; Part One covers what may be termed 'Adaptive Behaviour' while Part Two gives a profile of 'Maladaptive Behaviour'. If we look at the Profile Summary Part One (Figure 3.3) we can see that Geoff scores high on Physical Development (II) and low on all of the others, especially Independent Functioning, (I), Language Development (IV), Self Direction (VIII) and Socialisation (X). These latter areas were clearly sites requiring nursing interventions.

If we turn to the Profile Summary Part Two (Figure 3.4), which covers Maladaptive Behavior, we can see that Geoff scores high on all items except Psychological Disturbance with especially

Fig. 3.2 Data summary sheet 2

DATA SUMMARY SHEET PART TWO

I. VIOLENT AND DESTRUCTIVE BEHAVIOR	4	I
II. ANTISOCIAL BEHAVIOR	4	II
III. REBELLIOUS BEHAVIOR	4	III
IV. UNTRUSTWORTHY BEHAVIOR	2	IV
V. WITHDRAWAL	14	V
VI. STEREOTYPED BEHAVIOR AND ODD MANNERISMS	8	VI
VII. INAPPROPRIATE INTERPERSONAL MANNERS	6	VII
VIII. UNACCEPTABLE VOCAL HABITS	0	VIII
IX. UNACCEPTABLE OR ECCENTRIC HABITS	4	IX
X. SELF-ABUSIVE BEHAVIOR	0	X
XI. HYPERACTIVE TENDENCIES	3	XI
XII. SEXUALLY ABERRANT BEHAVIOR	4	XII
XIII. PSYCHOLOGICAL DISTURBANCES	I	XIII
XIV. USE OF MEDICATIONS	2	XIV

Fig. 3.3   ABS Profile Summary Part One

Name _Geoff W_
Age _24_
Sex _M_
Date of Administration _3/2/86_

PROFILE SUMMARY
AAMD ADAPTIVE BEHAVIOR SCALE PART ONE

Deciles	I Independent Functioning	II Physical Development	III Economic Activity	IV Language Development	V Numbers and Time	VI Domestic Activity	VII Vocational Activity	VIII Self-Direction	IX Responsibility	X Socialization
D9 (90)										
D8 (80)										
D7 (70)										
D6 (60)										
D5 (50)		52								
D4 (40)										
D3 (30)										
D2 (20)			25				21		21	
D1 (10)					15	14				
	5			5				1		1
Attained Scores	36	22	0	2	0	0	0	0	0	0

high scores on Withdrawal (V) (surprisingly), Stereotypic Behavior (VI) and Inappropriate Interpersonal Manners (VII), several others following closely behind.

In view of such an array of negative behaviours (Figure 3.4) it was even more important to match Geoff's weaknesses by as many strengths as possible. A long list could easily have been drawn up of negative behaviours, but instead, positive behavioural goals were set. The battery of information gathered from other members of the care team and my own diary of clinical notes acted as a basis for drawing up a set of care plans. As the overall philosophy of care was primarily a social skills approach it was decided to draw up a Primary Assessment Profile (Figure 3.5) based on an extention of those features earlier identified by the ABS and PAC.

As can be seen, this profile is intended to summarise the information previously gathered,

Fig. 3.4 ABS Profile Summary Part Two

Name _Geoff N_
Age _24_
Sex _M_
Date of Administration _3/2/86_

in a form that is accessible to those concerned with Geoff's care. Most of this information is self-explanatory but will be covered in discussion of Geoff's strengths and weaknesses and the resulting nursing problems and care plans.

Geoff's strengths were summarised as follows:

1. Assessment showed that his physical development was good, and hence that there was no reason—except his own motivation—why further skills could not be developed.

2. His general level of self-help skills was also good considering the dependence of other residents in the ward. In view of the other many problems that he had, I felt that this was of a relatively low priority.

3. He had a likeable personality; this was an asset because it attracts other staff to work with him.

Fig. 3.5 Primary Assessment Profile

NAME Geoff W.	WARD Oaks		DATE 10.2.86

ASSESSMENT STRATEGIES USED	PAC, ABS, CLINICAL DIARY

Self help

1. **Table skills** Is able to feed himself with a fork or spoon, as appropriate. If encouraged will hold a knife in his left hand but does not yet use it. Is learning to use a knife for spreading and cutting. Is able to pour himself a drink from a jug with reasonable care. Table behaviour is untidy and needs much encouragement.

2. **Washing** At the time of assessment Geoff will attempt to rub his face with a prepared flannel or towel. Needs encouragement to rub more than his lips. Resists cleaning teeth.

3. **Toileting** Is fully continent and able to take himself to the toilet without reminder, though does not use toilet paper. Adjustment of clothing afterwards is careless.

4. **Dressing** Able to dress and undress completely with encouragement but is unable to manage zips and buttons.

Language

1. **Receptive** Understanding of speech appears good, confined to single stage requests. Speech therapist thought that comprehension was largely situational. Very difficult to assess adequately.

2. **Expressive** Expressive language is confined to one or two immature vocalisations but no speech. He will take people to what he wants and gives many body language cues, but no executive signing.

Socialisation Geoff's social activities are confined to nursing staff and parents and are of a boisterous nature. He appears to recognise familiar people and usually greets them with a smile. He does not attempt to make contact with other residents and spends much of his time in stereotyped play on his own.

Occupation

1. **Gross motor skills** Geoff's physical development is normal: he is a healthy boisterous young man able to carry out the physical activities of the average two-year old.

2. **Fine motor skills** Fine motor skills are not highly developed, apparently through lack of practice stemming from a distinct lack of motivation.

3. **Play and understanding** Geoff's level of understanding appears to be confined to the 'here and now'. His play, when not stereotypic is that of a boisterous toddler, being interested in large, bright and noisy objects, preferably with plenty of movement involved.

4. **Self-amusement skills** Geoff's ability to amuse himself and to focus on play is not good. He is distractable and has a short attention span coupled to an apparent lack of motivation. When not being occupied he regularly engages in stereotypic play (15–25 min per hour), and periodically in open masturbation (2–3 times daily).

Personality incl. likes, dislikes and general behaviour Geoff's personality is generally a very happy and boisterous one. Fortunately, for one of so generous a build he is not at all aggressive. He will throw a temper tantrum occasionally when annoyed, but this is unusual. He is sometimes difficult to handle, but this is mainly due to his unwillingness to do things that he does not want to do and he is aware that he is stronger than most nursing staff. Tends to over-eat and is hence rather obese (15st 10 lb).

Fig. 3.5   (continued)

NAME Geoff W.	WARD Oaks	DATE 10.2.86

ASSESSMENT STRATEGIES USED   **PAC, ABS, CLINICAL DIARY**

Home contact   Parents are together and involved. Father comes to take him home from Friday evening to Monday morning every weekend, which Geoff looks forward to and thoroughly enjoys. His parents describe obsessive and manipulative behaviour while at home and that he slaps his ears if thwarted. Father takes him for long walks (15–20 miles) and consequently he arrives back at the ward exhausted for a day or so.

Current medication   1. Thioridazine 50 mg, three times daily.
2. Flurazepam 15 mg, at night when necessary.

Strengths   1. Physical development is good. There is no obvious reason why fine motor and self-help skills could not be developed further.
2. General level of self-help skills is good considering the character of the ward and the level of dependence of most of the other residents.
3. His personality is such that he is likeable.
4. His parents are still involved.

Weaknesses   1. Concentration is poor and attention span short. Motivation to learn new tasks is extremely low.
2. Receptive language is poor and executive language virtually non-existent making communication difficult.
3. His high level of energy and preference for stereotypic activities are resistant to change.
4. By dint of sheer size and strength he is able to avoid situations not to his liking.

Problem areas   1. Poor communication and social skills.
2. Preference for stereotypic activities.
3. Poor concentration and motivation.
4. Play skills poorly developed.
5. Open masturbation is socially undesirable.
6. Over-eating and obesity.
7. Level of activity varies over the week but remains problematical.
8. Parents' coping behaviour is at variance with that of the ward.

Comments   Many of the above problems are interlinked and related to Geoff's overall level of understanding.

4. His parents' continued involvement was a strength because potentially they were able to add a wider dimension to Geoff's life.

Geoff's weaknesses were summarised as follows:

1. His concentration and motivation to learn new tasks were poor. This was probably his greatest barrier to further learning and needed to be tackled.

2. His poor language skills made communication with him very difficult and was again a fundamental problem.

3. His overall level of energy was high and he had a preference for stereotypic play, e.g. twisting strips of cloth or string, distracting his attention from other learning activities.

4. His sheer size and weight made him difficult to handle at times and led to his labelling by staff as a 'problem'.

The planning of care

Although the above strengths and weaknesses do not directly lead to identification of nursing problems they are useful in maintaining an over-all view of Geoff that was balanced in terms of positive and negative aspects. From the overall assessment, and by using both objective and subjective criteria, Geoff's nursing problems as detailed on the Assessment Profile were now related to a series of care plans.

Care plan 1, (Figure 3.6), refers to Geoff's poor communication and social skills. This area was seen as fundamental to Geoff's subsequent social development and care, both to facilitate Geoff's feedback regarding his needs and de-sires, and for nursing staff to convey social approval and reinforcement. If Geoff remained indifferent to social intercourse, his behaviour modification would become the more difficult; perhaps even intractable.

My goal here was to find activities that included a sense of mutual enjoyment and so stimulate Geoff's social awareness, plus his need to communicate. This was a short-term goal which, when reached, would have supplied a fund of activities that could be used as part of a long-term goal to meet the same problem.

My intervention used three strategies in an experimental way which in practice were used in combination with each other.

1. 'Free play' situations were encouraged as the opportunity arose to develop Geoff's trust in me through mutual enjoyment of the activities.
2. 'Gross play' was employed (rough and tumble and the use of large play equipment) in an attempt to find activities that Geoff would enjoy for their own sake.
3. At the same time and throughout the day I encouraged any vocalisations that Geoff made, mirroring them and making the most of them while modelling speech by the use of controlled conversation.

This care plan was evaluated at the end of five weeks and it was noted that Geoff seemed to be making both vocal and behavioural responses. Geoff's father told me that he seemed calmer at

Fig. 3.6   Care plan 1

Name	Geoff W.	Date	13/2/86	Evaluation date	2/3/86	Short or long-term goal?	Short
Client problem		Nursing goal and planned intervention				Evaluation	
Social activity is avoided by Geoff and he shows little ability to communicate his wants		To find enjoyable activities which will stimulate Geoff's social awareness and skills 1. Using free-play situations develop a relationship based on trust and mutual enjoyment 2. Experiment with gross play situations in order to find activities which Geoff finds intrinsically enjoyable 3. Encourage vocalisations that may be prompted by such situations, using mirroring and modelling				This strategy appears to be pro-ducing promising results. Geoff's enjoyment is evident and he will often initiate games in a very simple way. He appears calmer for most of the time and is vocali-sing more and producing a wide variety of sounds. At home father reports a favourable change, Geoff being calmer and saying words, though one must be scep-tical about the latter. As results are so far good, this strategy should be continued as a long-term activity	

home and was making sounds that his parents interpreted as words.

Care plan 2 (Figure 3.7) refers to Geoff's preference for stereotypic activities, which typically consisted of laying on tables or work surfaces and rocking and twiddling braces or other similar objects and banging and mouthing plastic toys while striding up and down the room. While these were not intrinsically wrong they prevented him from more constructive activities and the learning of further skills. This behaviour was also labelled by the ward and training department staff as undesirable. My goal in this was the simple one of decreasing the frequency of Geoff's stereotypic play; the technique used as part of my interventive strategy was that of differential reinforcement of other behaviours, and can be seen in relation to the goal of care plans 3 and 4.

In simple terms, plenty of situations were provided in which Geoff could 'play' in a constructive way. I reinforced this behaviour by plenty of social and occasional material rewards while, at the same time, removing his twiddles and encouraging him to join in my activities. A full description of this technique can be found in Carr (1979). My evaluation at the end of the five weeks was that Geoff's attention to constructive activities had increased from a few minutes to as much as 35 minutes in the right circumstances. He was markedly better in this while attending the training department than on the ward, where the strategy could have been more rigorously applied.

The problem which care plan 3 (Figure 3.8) attempted to meet was Geoff's poor concentration and motivation; my goal in this case was to find reinforcers which could then be used to build up his concentration span. My planned strategy in this case was:

1. To find a range of toys and equipment that Geoff was able to cope with. I found, for instance, that puzzles of any kind that presented a broken image were meaningless to him but that he coped well with inset puzzles that presented whole images.
2. To systematically use a variety of different possible reinforcers such as dolly mixtures, fragments of biscuits and crisps, flavoured powders such as sherbet and lemonade powders, and listening to music.

Fig. 3.7   Care plan 2

Name	Geoff W.	Date	13/2/86	Evaluation date	2/3/86	Short or long-term goal?	Long

Client problem	Nursing goal and planned intervention	Evaluation
Fixated at stereotypic play level and limited in his scope for emotional and behavioural expression	To decrease the frequency of stereotypic play and encourage Geoff to further his potential to relate more closely to his social environment via play activity 1. Provide plenty of situations for Geoff to play in a constructive way 2. Encourage constructive play using social and occasionally material rewards 3. Discourage stereotypies by verbal means and when practical take away the objects with which Geoff is playing stereotypically	Geoff can now be constructively occupied for about 35 min, depending on situation and time of the week, though is markedly better in the training department than on the ward It is recommended that this strategy be continued and that it be more rigorously applied on the ward

Fig. 3.8   Care plan 3

Name	Geoff W.	Date	13/2/86	Evaluation date	2/3/86	Short or long-term goal?	Short
Client problem		Nursing goal and planned intervention				Evaluation	
Poor concentration and motivation		To find suitable reinforcers with which to build up concentration using external motivation 1. To find a variety of simple toys which Geoff is intellectually able to master 2. Using a variety of possible reinforcers, use these systematically in order to discover if any of them are sufficiently powerful to motivate Geoff				Geoff appears to work well for sherbet and flavoured powders applied to his tongue by the nurse's finger Toys which he can master in this situation are simple inset puzzles which do not require symbolic imagery and posting boxes of various degrees of difficulty	

I was able to evaluate this care plan after one week because it quickly became obvious that Geoff's motivation markedly improved when he knew that sherbet would be forthcoming. The care plan was therefore ruled through and care plan 4 substituted in its place (Figure 3.9).

Care plan 4 was drawn up to attempt to meet two related problems. These were:

1. Again Geoff's poor concentration and motivation.
2. Geoff's poorly developed play (I should more properly say self-amusement) skills.

The overall goal of this care plan was to increase Geoff's concentration and 'play' skills using external motivation, with the long-term inten-

Fig. 3.9   Care plan 4

Name	Geoff W.	Date	19/2/86	Evaluation date	2/3/86	Short or long term goal?	Long
Client problem		Nursing goal and planned intervention				Evaluation	
(a) Poor concentration and motivation (b) Poorly developed play skills		To increase Geoff's concentration span and skills in order that acceptable toys may gain an intrinsic interest for him 1. Use a range of both familiar and new toys making a note of any that seem popular 2. Encourage Geoff to play with the toys in an appropriate way, giving plenty of social reward and occasional reinforcements using sherbet and flavoured powders on a variable reinforcement schedule				Geoff will now concentrate and play constructively at the table for up to 35 min using praise and fizzy-powder reinforcers. He performs well on inset puzzles and posting puzzles and appears to be finding intrinsic pleasure in a simple posting box with a door and key. It is recommended that this strategy be continued while attempting to broaden Geoff's scope	

tion that he would begin to develop skills of self-amusement other than stereotypes and masturbation.

To this end, activities were designed to attract Geoff's attention, with especial emphasis on toys that were familiar and used every day; a constant look-out was kept for fresh equipment, be it begged or borrowed from other departments. Geoff was given plenty of encouragement to use these in an appropriate way, given praise, and invited into ongoing activity that interested him. I also used a range of flavoured powders—on a variable reinforcement schedule basis—by dipping the end of my finger into the powder and applying it to the tip of Geoff's tongue. In view of the possibly obsessive aspect of Geoff's personality, care was taken to keep the choice of powder random and to make the reinforcement intervals random. This seemed to work well, for although the powders had an obvious motivating power, Geoff did not 'hover' looking for the next reinforcement 'fix' in the way one often observes in other training programs.

At the end of the five-week period Geoff would play for periods of up to 35 minutes. I was also able to note that he was beginning to find intrinsic pleasure in a certain posting box which used simple shapes and bright colours, with a door which opened via a large key. He would actively seek this toy out and spend several minutes playing with it without needing my encouragement. His enjoyment was apparent from his smiling face. This care plan was a long-term one, and so I concluded my evaluation by recommending its continuation. If the approach is right, results should be evident within one week when caring for all but the most profoundly handicapped.

Care plan 5 (Figure 3.10) was an attempt to provide a constructive solution to Geoff's open masturbation which, although not a problem in itself, was socially unacceptable and a problem for Geoff in that such behaviour limited the choice of future placements.

My goal in this case was that Geoff should learn to masturbate only in an acceptable setting.

Fig. 3.10   Care plan 5

Name	Geoff W.	Date	13/2/86	Evaluation date	2/3/86	Short or long-term goal?	Short
Client problem		**Nursing goal and planned intervention**				**Evaluation**	
Open masturbation (being socially unacceptable)		That Geoff should be discouraged from masturbating in the day area. If persistent should be taken by the hand to an area of privacy 1. If Geoff is seen with his hand in the front of his trousers he should be told, 'Take your hand out Geoff' 2. If Geoff is seen openly masturbating he should be told, 'Put it away Geoff' 3. If Geoff persists in masturbating he should be encouraged to find a more appropriate place, i.e. a vacant dormitory, the bathroom or a secluded part of the garden (site to be varied to avoid the act of masturbation becoming linked with any one specific place)				It has been noted that Geoff will usually only masturbate while on the ward, and then only when bored. It is not seen while he is being constructively occupied. It seems essential to provide plenty of activities for Geoff in order for him to be well occupied	

The bedroom, although being the obvious choice, was not used as Geoff shared an open plan bedroom with five other men; this area was therefore inappropriate. The intervention used was loosely based on differential reinforcement and took the form of three stages:

1. If Geoff was seen with his hand in the front of his trousers he was told simply to take his hand out.
2. If he was seen openly masturbating he was told simply to put his penis away.
3. If Geoff continued to masturbate he was encouraged to enter an area where he might meet his sexual needs in privacy.

In all cases, the nurse's tone of voice was not loaded with disapproval and Geoff was only asked to stop what he was doing. This precluded the possibility that Geoff masturbated for attention rather than his own more immediate gratification.

The reinforcement of other behaviours is covered by Care plan 2 which is borne out by my evaluation notes at the end of the initial five-week period when I observed that Geoff appeared to masturbate more frequently while on the ward. This seemed coupled more to boredom than anything else. I concluded that it seemed essential to provide Geoff with plenty of activities in order to help him more meaningfully occupy his time.

Care plan 6 (Figure 3.11) was drawn up because Geoff was very much overweight, with a large flabby paunch. This was a problem because his clothes were beginning no longer to fit him and he had difficulty in fastening his trousers over his very large tummy. My goal was therefore to reduce his overall weight and to reduce his paunch so he would have less difficulty with his clothes. My intention was to consult his parents about this and, with their agreement, replace foods in Geoff's diet having a high carbohydrate content with more green vegetables or fresh fruit.

To my consternation, however, Geoff's parents emphatically told me that one of Geoff's great pleasures in life was eating, and that if the hospital reduced his food intake they would compensate by giving him more at home (he already ate enormous amounts of food while at home).

In spite of my reassurances that Geoff would not be eating less food but merely more healthy food, they were adamant. I felt that their attitude spoke volumes about their relationship with the ward staff and with the hospital in general, borne

Fig. 3.11   Care plan 6

Name	Geoff W.	Date	13/2/86	Evaluation date	2/3/86	Short or long-term goal?	Short
Client problem			Nursing goal and planned intervention			Evaluation	
Geoff is overweight with a flabby paunch. His clothes no longer fit properly; present weight 15 st 10 lb			To reduce Geoff's overall weight with consequent reduction in paunch so that his trousers will fit properly: Target weight, 12 st 7 lb, consistent with height and frame With parents' permission, foods with a high carbohydrate content should be reduced and replaced with more green vegetables or fresh fruit			This goal has not been met because Geoff's parents emphatically state that if the ward reduce his food intake, they will compensate by giving him even more at weekends This is indicative of a deep-seated gap between the hospital and Geoff's parents. Perhaps more help needs to be carried out in this area as a priority		

out by their rather formal relationship with the staff and reluctance to communicate with them.

Care plan 7 (Figure 3.12) is a long-term plan and relates to Geoff's level of activity, which varied over the week, but remained a problem. As part of Geoff's weekend activities his parents would take him for walks of between fifteeen and twenty miles on a Friday evening, Saturday and Sunday. This was partly because Geoff genuinely enjoys long walks and partly to give him a legitimate means of using up his large store of energy. It was usual for him to return to the ward on Monday morning barely able to keep his eyes open and therefore unable to take part in any constructive activities. As the week progressed however, his energy level would rise until on Fridays he was very 'high' and too energetic to concentrate on constructive activities for long.

The goal in this case was to even out the level of activity over the week so that Geoff would pose less of a problem to both ward staff and his parents. Intervention took three stages:

1. I discussed the problem with Geoff's father and told him of my proposed plans as detailed in (2) and (3).

2. During the early part of the week when Geoff was drowsy I would allow him to recuperate while at the same time encouraging as much constructive activity as possible.

3. Towards the end of the week, when Geoff's energy level became a problem, I would provide opportunities for him to expend this energy in lengthy walks of five miles or so which could be taken with a number of other residents and in other active play situations.

Such an approach appeared to work well, as noted in the evaluation at the end of the five-week period. Geoff's father told me that he was calmer and more manageable at home and did not need to be taken for such long walks. Father was obviously very pleased by this as it constituted a meaningful advance for the family and helped to bridge the gap between ward and home. Geoff returned on Monday mornings less sleepy and more ready to join in with activities. The walks were a source of enjoyment to Geoff and were often a time when he vocalised most. As this strategy was evidently successful, I felt that it should be continued as part of a long-term care plan.

Fig. 3.12 Care plan 7

Name	Geoff W.	Date	13/2/86	Evaluation date	2/3/86	Short or long-term goal?	Long
Client problem			Nursing goal and planned intervention			Evaluation	

Client problem	Nursing goal and planned intervention	Evaluation
Geoff's energy is low early in the week (Mon.–Wed.) and very high later in the week (Thur.–Sun.) so causing disturbances of attention and sleep	To even out the differential in activity level from Monday to Friday 1. Parents and the clinical team discuss this problem in order to formulate a strategy acceptable to both parties 2. During the early part of the week when Geoff is drowsy, he should be allowed quiet activities in order to recuperate while at the same time stimulating him sufficiently 3. Towards the end of the week, when overactivity is the problem, Geoff should be given ample opportunity to use his energy in a legitimate way	This approach appears to be valid as father reports that Geoff is more manageable and calmer at home. On the ward, the activity differential is less marked over the week. Geoff is less drowsy on Monday and Tuesday, but still becomes very high on Friday. In view of the encouraging results so far, it is recommended that this strategy be continued

The last care plan in the series, care plan 8 (Figure 3.13) related to the obvious gap between Geoff's parents' strategy, the philosophy of care, and the rôle of the ward. I felt that to embark on a programme of therapy with the family that could not be sustained would have been ethically inexcusable. I therefore postponed this goal to a later date.

The goal in this case was to develop coping strategies between home and the ward that would provide a more continuous pattern of care throughout the week. I felt that this goal could have been met in two ways:

1. That Geoff's parents and the clinical team should discuss openly and on equal footing their ideas of the family's needs, and attempt to develop a plan of care that would be of mutual concern and benefit. This was essential if Geoff's parents were not to feel alienated from his life in the hospital.
2. At the same time, Geoff's parents should be sensitively helped, and encouraged to accept professional support in changing Geoff's behaviour at home, which from their own

reports they often found very disturbing and disruptive. Simply, the family unit was also to be cared for, besides Geoff.

Re-appraisal of the afore-mentioned model of care: insights towards a fresh approach for mentally handicapped people

Although the model described so far was workable and was not without success, after some discussion and further re-examination, a number of shortcomings became evident. These were:

1. The approach was not needs-driven; that is, nursing problems did not necessarily derive from the client's needs but rather from a complex mixture of objective and subjective observations (PAC/ABS diary observations).
2. The care was too narrow in its approach; it worked for a physically able person whose needs were mainly social, but I doubted its

Fig. 3.13　Care plan 8

Name	Geoff W.	Date	13/2/86	Evaluation date	2/3/86	Short or long-term goal?	Long
Client problem			**Nursing goal and planned intervention**			**Evaluation**	
Parents' coping behaviour is at variance with that of the ward			To develop coping strategies between home and ward that will provide a more continuous pattern of care throughout the week 1. Parents and the clinical team should meet to discuss openly and on equal footing their perceptions of Geoff's needs and to isolate areas which are of *mutual* concern 2. Geoff's parents should be introduced to the idea of allowing professional input into the home situation in order to help them to develop adaptive coping strategies			This is a long-standing difficulty which has been a problem for many years and is unlikely to be resolved in a few weeks. Geoff's parents have so far strongly resisted all efforts at intervention by ward or community staff; historically, the ward and family have seen each other as 'threatening' and withdrawn from communication. This goal should be continued as a long-term objective	

suitability and usefulness with, for instance, a person with multiple handicaps, including cerebral palsy. There was obviously a need to develop, if possible, a model that was wide in its compass and could be used with all mentally handicapped people.

3. The approach did not help the nurse to pinpoint nursing problems and did not lead logically to the development of care plans. I felt that too much of my previous work was subjective, personal and could not easily be transferred for use by other nursing staff without a fairly long spell of orientation; it needed to be made less cumbersome.

These three points then, led to the search for a second, more developed perspective based on wider principles of client care. With the help of my colleagues I therefore set out to make a list of the needs of mentally handicapped people that were not specific to one client group, and that applied equally to those in hospital and community. From an initial list of over sixty items which were correlated into groups or categories, we finally arrived at a list of twelve living needs or activities of daily living—to borrow Roper's terminology—that reflected the nature of mentally handicapped people (Figure 3.14).

The subheadings in Figure 3.14 will now be examined in closer detail.

1. Communicating
This includes the verbal, non-verbal, receptive and expressive needs of the person and assessment aims to identify particular problems with communicating that a client might have.

2. Psychological needs
This was an area in little evidence in the previous model, and yet, is of obvious importance. Areas for assessment under this heading are self concept—does the person have any knowledge of 'self', of 'me-ness' and, linked to this, the concept of self-esteem or self-worth? Sexuality was an area that I considered should be included under the heading of psychological needs rather than being a need in itself. This is not to denigrate its importance (which has long been ignored in the field of mental handicap) but to integrate it with other related needs. Sexuality is not just about the sexual function but about being a man or being a woman, behaving in a way that is appropriate, as well as knowledge of one's body and its way of working. Sexuality is therefore in my view related to areas of self-concept and self-worth. Love and belongingness, friendship and warmth are also needs that we

Fig. 3.14 Activities of living

1. *Communicating*	verbal, non verbal	7. *Physiological needs*	breathing, eliminating epilepsy
2. *Psychological needs*	self-concept, self-esteem, sexuality, love and belonging-ness, dying	8. *Work and leisure*	meaningful occupation, education, leisure, worship/spiritual
3. *Eating and drinking*	ability for self-care, need for special techniques, need for special aids	9. *Personal care*	hygiene, clothing/dressing, toilet, motivation to self-care
4. *Social skills*	interpersonal skills, social norms, social mixing	10. *Safety needs*	potential of risk to self/others, self-mutilation, aggression, wandering, knowledge of danger
5. *Family and friends*	degree of involvement, pattern of home life, significant others		
6. *Mobility*	fine/gross motor skills, need for aids, need for therapy	11. *Sleep and rest*	sleep/waking pattern, length of sleep, nocturnal activities
		12. *Perception*	seeing, hearing, sensitivity, other sensory handicaps

have in varying proportion according to our personality and our psychological development, and lastly dying. It may seem peculiar that I have included dying under this heading, but I felt that the physical needs of the dying person were (or should be) both evident and included under the physical needs. The psychological needs of the dying person and indeed the bereaved person are sometimes forgotten, especially when that person is mentally handicapped. They should therefore be properly included under this heading.

3. Eating and drinking

This covers a person's ability to manage eating and drinking independently, their ability to physically manipulate the utensils and the relevant parts of their own body, their need for physical help and training, special aids and utensils to help them to be independent, and the need, especially with physically handicapped people, for special techniques in relation to feeding in order to overcome tongue thirst, bite reflex and so on. Not to be forgotten here are any food idiosyncracies or special diet that the person may need, and a note of any food and drink likes and dislikes that the person may have.

4. Social skills

Here social skills are addressed and understood in the true sense of the word—as those various interpersonal skills that a person needs in order to live in harmony with others. This includes adjustment to social norms, being able to adjust to the social needs of others and social mixing; being able to make friends and join in with social activities.

5. Family and friends

These are not really a need, and yet, are more inclusive than just affiliative needs. We considered that there was a need to have full information about the family—their degree of involvement, the pattern of home life and the expectations they make of each other. This is especially important where we work in partnership with families. Also important are those 'significant others', people who are close to the client and yet are not directly members of the family. We might include here members of staff who have a particularly close relationship with the client, people who live in the home or hospital with whom the client has a close relationship, and people like voluntary workers who have a special involvement.

6. Mobility

As this is an area which commonly presents problems to the mentally handicapped person, I considered it to merit a category of its own. The term mobility is however to be liberally interpreted and is intended to cover both gross and fine motor skills. Gross motor skills include the skills of balance, sitting, creeping, crawling and walking and the control of movements of whole limbs. Fine motor skills are the finer movements of the hands needed for the skills of picking up, grasping, manipulating and letting go. Here we also need to assess the need for special aids to independence, including the use (especially independently if possible) of wheelchairs, special seating and other mobility aids, and the need for special therapy. As with other areas, there may be a need for the involvement of other professionals, but the problem and the consequent care-need would be included as part of a comprehensive assessment.

7. Physiological needs

This area really covers all other physical needs not covered by mobility. Here I would include breathing, the risk of pressure sores, eliminating (often a problem for physically handicapped people) the physical risks encountered as part of a person's epilepsy and other nursing demands of a medical nature that the person may make.

8. Work and leisure

Heading the list in this category is the need for meaningful occupation. This includes educational needs (whether a client is of school age or not); the need for work of a meaningful kind, and the need for a programme of leisure that ensures that a person's recreational needs are fully met. I have also included here the person's worship and spiritual needs as they form an integral part of some people's lives.

9. *Personal care*

This really includes what are often called the self-help skills and covers washing, cleaning of teeth, dressing, choosing suitable clothes, self-toileting, housekeeping skills and generating a person's motivation to care for himself.

10. *Safety needs*

This is a very wide category, and is intended to cover a person's potential to place himself and others at risk via aggression or self-harm, the consequences of harm from any medical condition (i.e. epilepsy), the likelihood of wandering and losing oneself, danger from traffic, the person's knowledge of dangers in the environment such as fire, boiling water, deep water, traffic and various moral dangers such as sexual exploitation or alcohol abuse.

11. *Sleep and rest*

This includes the person's pattern of sleeping and waking, the usual length of sleep, how and where the person likes to sleep and any preparations that are normally made prior to sleeping and waking. Nocturnal activities are taken to mean the kind of activities that the person may indulge in at night such as wandering, coming into parents' bed and so on.

12. *Perception*

This area is intended for the assessment and identification of perceptual problems such as blindness or partial sight—including the need for spectacles and other visual aids, deafness or the need for aids to enable the betterment of various 'sensation tones' or 'hypersensitivity'. As the incidence of perceptual problems is much higher in mentally handicapped people than the general population, one should always suspect these, especially with new clients suffering from multiple handicaps.

Each person has his or her own peculiar needs which cannot necessarily be covered by even the most exhaustive assessments, however well planned. The model suggested depends on the skill of each nurse to adapt creatively the assessment to address the needs and individual characteristics of their client.

This particular model of assessment is not intended to replace those better-known assessment tools used in the field of mental handicap, but to complement these, as an additional means of gathering information about the handicapped person. My suggested format for the use of this approach bears a number of similarities to the one used earlier. A suggested format for a simple understanding of the twelve assessments is offered in Figure 3.15 where a front sheet is shown. It contains the minimum of information necessary for identification of the file and the person to whom it relates. Many nursing process record forms duplicate much of the information in the client's clinical folder or its equivalent. This is unnecessary and merely adds to the amount of paperwork which dogs the modern nurse and forms one of the main objections to the use of a nursing process approach. The space for a photograph was suggested by staff within my own hospital, and serves as a form of positive identification for newcomers to the ward. In ideal circumstances this should be unnecessary, and I suspect may prove somewhat redundant in practice. The greater part of this front sheet is taken assessment together with a scale of dependence/independence for each one. This is intended for completion after the main part of assessment has been carried out as an aid to identification of areas providing nursing problems. I will not suggest assessment methods, nor ways of recording these, for this is for each individual nurse to decide in the light of her own establishment's policy. What does concern me is making the information as clear and precise as possible, and Figure 3.15 is my best effort so far. There are three separate ways in which the continuum can be filled. One way is to place the client by comparison with normal development, i.e. non-handicapped people of his own age, but this is only of real use with the least handicapped client. The second way is to compare him with the average attainment of those people with whom he resides. Though this may prove useful my own preference is to use the scale as a comparison with other skills the subject has, so that the nurse is able to gain an idea of the comparative urgency for interventive work. This

Figure. 3.15   Care plan, suggested front sheet

Name			
Address			Photograph
D.O.B.		D.O.A.	
Ass. date		Signed	
Ward			

	Dependence	Independence
Eating and drinking		
Personal care		
Mobility		
Physiological needs		
Sleep and rest		
Communicating		
Perceiving		
Psychological needs		
Social skills		
Work and leisure		
Safety needs		
Family and friends		

technique has been adapted largely from Roper's model. Figure 3.16 shows a suggested format for recording this information so that post-assessment strengths, weaknesses, and problematic nursing areas can be seen at a glance.

Client-centred problems and care goals may be explored and evaluated on the suggested ongoing data sheet (Figure 3.17). As care needs change a fresh sheet would be commenced as illustrated in the earlier care study.

Fig. 3.16 Data record sheet: Nursing process secondary level assessment

Name			Ward		
Assessment dates			Assessors' initials		
Assessment tools used					
Strengths					
Weaknesses					
Identified nursing problems (not in order of precedence)					

The advantage of using a fresh sheet for each care plan is that when evaluated it can be placed at the back of the client's nursing process folder and replaced by its successor. This obviates the need to search through a list of care plans for ones that are currently in use.

This 'improved' assessment format has been piloted in the hospital where I work and has proved itself to be well suited to the needs of our clients. It has been successfully used by both qualified staff and student nurses preparing for their nursing care assessment. This is not to say that it is without flaws; I would expect it to continue to evolve over the next few years before reaching anywhere near its final form.

It is only by analysis of what we do that we will raise the level of our art and the status of our profession. We need to evolve models that truly reflect the needs of our clients. The approach suggested is one way—if it attracts you go out and use it, not slavishly, but rather with an eye to its possible improvement and adaptation for those clients for whom you care.

I started out looking for a model to help me in my nursing and ended up with the client's nursing needs suggesting a model to me. I hope that your enquiry will be as professionally enriching as my own.

Critique

The amount of paperwork and plan revision demonstrated by the mode of care suggested by this

Fig. 3.17   Ongoing data sheet

Name	Date	Evaluation date		Short or long-term goal?
Client problem	Nursing goal and planned intervention			Evaluation

chapter, although thorough, might be perceived by the reader as excessive. The author recognises the importance of the time spent on assessment and sees this as being essential for subsequent care efficiency. But, were the various social assessment charts any more meaningful than straightforward nursing observations?

Though teamwork is stated as an important requisite of care, little of this is evident in the text.

The author's position within the clinical area sheds light on the above; he was himself new to the ward and had to rely upon the goodwill of others; his choice of assessment tools was similarly a concession to ward practice. It would have caused greater alienation to introduce new tools or to stipulate a teamwork approach before the relevance of either had been successfully demonstrated to his colleagues.

Less understandable is the rationale to forsake established nursing models for the troublesome process of refining an original one; conversely, much personal development can occur from such an approach.

Paul Barber

Salient questions

1. Has the author made his approach to the nursing process over-complex?
2. Are the assessment tools used in the text central or superfluous to the care described?
3. How might the family have been more successfully involved in care planning?
4. What were the gains in evolving an idiosyncratic model of care?
5. Which nursing models could have been fruitfully employed to enhance care?
6. Did the form of the nursing model complement the concept of normalisation, and if you feel it did not, what other strategy might have replaced the one illustrated?
7. Is the model suggested by the author significantly different to merit further development?

References

Aggleton P & Chalmers H   1984   Models and theories: defining the terms, *Nursing Times*, (September 5), 24–28.

Bailey RD 1982 *Therapeutic Nursing for the Mentally Handicapped*, Oxford University Press, Oxford.

Bowness S & Zadik TD 1981 Implementing the nursing process at a unit for mentally handicapped children, *Nursing Times*, (April 16), 695–696.

Carr J 1979 *Helping Your Handicapped Child*, Penguin, Harmondsworth.

Crow J 1979 In: Kratz C (ed), *The Nursing Process*, Baillière Tindall, London.

Green C 1984 The application of the nursing process to mental handicap in a hospital setting, *Nurse Education Today*, 127–131.

Gunzburg HC 1973 *Social Competence and Mental Handicap* (2nd edition), Baillière Tindall, London.

Gunzburg HC 1977 *PAC Manual Vol. 1*, SEFA, London.

Leslie FA & Shiells E 1981 The nursing process related to mental handicap care. *Nursing Times*, (July), 1169–1174.

Nihira K *et al.* 1975 *AAMD Adaptive Behavior Scale* (1974 Revision). American Association on Mental Deficiency, Washington.

Roper N *et al.* 1980 *The Elements of Nursing*, Churchill Livingstone, Edinburgh.

Roy SC 1970 Adaption: a conceptual framework for nursing, *Nursing Outlook*, **18**, 42–45.

Samy T 1983a Structured assessment, *Nursing Mirror*, November 23, Mental Health Forum 10, i–v.

Samy T 1983b Making the most of his days, *Nursing Mirror*, November 23, Mental Health Forum 10, x–xii.

4

Understanding the nature of a therapeutic relationship in behavioural programming— a behaviour therapy perspective

Paul Barber and Martin Brown

Summary

The following chapter combines two main themes: the rôle of the behaviour therapist and the relational model of Hildegard Peplau. Both these approaches have contrasting—though the authors contend complementary—qualities and a dialogue is pursued throughout the care study which compares and contrasts the philosophy of each.

Behavioural rationale is explained, both in its historical and current context, and a relationship drawn between 'educating the behaviour' and 'developing the person' of the client via the medium of the nurse–patient relationship. Attempts are made to link the 'scientific methodology' of behaviourism to the 'interpersonal appreciation' of the chosen nursing model. The illustrative care study relates to a middle-aged client who has recently been transferred from a large institution to a small community home, and examines nursing interventions to correct his reactive behaviour disturbance. Throughout this study 'behavioural stages' and 'relationship phases' are introduced into the care picture and related to therapeutic nursing practice.

Paul Barber

Introduction

Behaviourism is historically associated with the work of Pavlov, Skinner and Watson, whose theories of learning attempt to show that com- mon principles are involved in the way we learn to behave, and that these same principles may be therapeutically manipulated to modify inappro- priate responses. Watson (1924) believed that only simple psychological reflexes were inheri- ted, all else being a product of learning:

> Give me a dozen healthy infants, well-formed, and my own specified world to bring them up in and I'll guarantee to take any one at random and train him to become any kind of specialist I might select— doctor, lawyer, artist, merchant, chief, and yes, even a beggar-man and thief, regardless of his talents, penchants, abilities, vocations, and race of his ancestors.
>
> (Watson, 1924)

The above viewpoint was supported by the work of Pavlov who demonstrated—in his now fam- ous experiment—that a dog could be trained to salivate merely at the sound of a bell previously associated with feeding; everything, seemingly, could be learnt. Skinner further extended this rationale of 'reflex conditioning' to include the 'creation of a Utopian society'—in his novel *Walden Two* (1948), 'speech' in his study *Verbal Behaviour* (1957) and in later works as a vehicle to 'put right all the wrongs of society'—*Beyond Freedom and Dignity* (1971) (see Stevanson, 1974, for a fuller description of Skinner's works).

Skinner dismissed all inner workings of the mind as of no explanatory value. He applied the findings of laboratory-animal experiments to explain human response. In the raw, Skinner's orientation is far from therapeutic in the traditional sense—he places little value upon feelings, personal choice, self-actualisation or other humanistic concepts. Thankfully behaviourism has evolved in directions other than those dictated by Skinner.

The work of Bandura in the 1950s and 1960s with regard to 'social learning theory' began to make more human the traditional cold mechanistic view of behaviourism. Bandura's Social Learning Model views abnormal behaviour as the result of faulty learning in the course of growing up; conversely, re-education may be enacted to solicit normal adjustment. In this perspective an individual's expectations gain recognition as moderators of behaviour. Therapeutically, client involvement desirable for re-education is best achieved through co-operative effort. Indeed, clients may come to direct their own therapy, taking the initiative to progress along avenues they suggest at a pace they feel most comfortable, little-by-little gaining mastery over those problems before them while coming to appreciate that efficient performance is the result of their own efforts.

In the 1970s, Mahoney (1974) and Meichenbaum (1975) began to look at the thinking processes involved in behaviour, and how, if these could be directly altered or modified, we could change the way that clients behaved. This is a far cry from Skinner, for here we are entering the 'black-box' of the mind and directly addressing the inner workings of individuals.

Ellis (1962) and Beck (1976) complement this approach, arguing that disturbed behaviour results from 'thinking errors' which in turn result from 'dysfunctional belief systems'. In mental handicap the above may be complicated by institutional living, the absence of suitable rôle models and isolation from the community.

Recently, Barker has drawn attention to the need for nurses to more fully appreciate the implications of using a behavioural approach and to answer the following questions prior to intervention:

— what is the nature of the problem?
— what should be the final treatment goals?
— when can treatment begin?
— how should the programme be organised?
— which change techniques would be appropriate?
— how should the programme be evaluated?
— will the programme raise any ethical dilemmas?

(Barker, 1982)

These questions will be returned to later in the care example of this chapter, where they are used to shape the assessment and review process prior to nursing intervention.

The connections between nursing and behaviour therapy are well documented elsewhere by Barker (1982, 1985), McPherson *et al.* (1978) and Marks *et al.* (1977). Essentially, they involve the education of nurses to utilise behavioural techniques within a wide range of psychiatric problems. According to Kazdim and Wilson (1978) behaviour therapy involves:

— a psychological model of nursing behaviour that differs from intrapsychic, psychodynamic or quasi-disease models of mental disorder;
— a commitment to scientific method, measurement and evaluation.

Though nursing action has often been effective it has rarely been scientific, with the consequence that nurses have been unable to share with their colleagues—and other care professionals—a 'therapeutic rationale'. Behaviour therapy fills this gap, and offers a psychological model that pre-supposes that behaviour is learned and can be unlearned or altered; and so provides a rationale for nursing action.

Child (1981) when discussing learning, says:

The basic premise is that learning occurs whenever one adapts new, or modifies existing behaviour patterns in a way that has some influence on future performance or attitudes.

Thus we could say a client had 'learned' to feed himself, or 'learned' to dress himself or 'learned' to socialise. This linking of nursing and behaviourism means that solutions to problems may become more pragmatic, more related to the individual's needs and wants and less fixed to theoretical dogma. By focusing upon the 'process' of therapy, rather than a description of its theoretical base, nurses are able to alter previously intractable behaviours.

Peggy Griffiths (1985) describes the behavioural management of a mentally handicapped woman with bathing and eating problems; similarly the treatment of a client with chronic pain is reported upon by William Harkin (1985) such is the currency and applicability of the behavioural approach.

Many clients in the field of mental handicap have multiple problems: physical deficits often go hand-in-hand with psycho-social dysfunctions and occasionally, with ensuing psychiatric disorders such as depressions, anxiety responses and obsessional behaviours. Such is the range of the behavioural model it may be used to address all of these. But, in all cases, success or failure depends upon the quality of the nurse's intervention and its appropriateness.

The behaviourist training model suggested by McFall (1976) concerns itself with two basic behaviour phenomena—excess and deficit. In behavioural excess, too much behaviour has been learned, for instance when a resident repeatedly visits the toilet and follows the sequence of behaviour associated with micturition and defaecation—even with no result, or when a client says repeatedly 'How do you do' to each and every person endlessly.

Deficits of behaviour are likewise easily identified—as when dressing, eating or social skills are obviously lacking. In both cases, the excess or deficit severely disrupts the individual's capacity to function independently—or simply to enjoy life. But, before we proceed a caution is necessary; there are several ethical issues raised by nurses using a behavioural approach. These are summarised in the following questions:

—How may we decide when behaviour is or isn't appropriate?
—How may we prevent the value judgements we cannot avoid making about other people affecting the outcomes of nursing?

—How may we avoid interference with the individual's right to choose to do as they wish?

There are no easy answers to the above—if there are any answers at all; but a partial answer could be suggested if the nurse is attuned to the client's needs and stays awake to the interpersonal process they both share, that is, stays self and interpersonally aware. Before we investigate the possibility of this we had better pursue a little further the behavioural model, and concentrate on the processes it involves. Broadly, there are four stages:

1. Systematic measurement and assessment of the presenting problems.
2. Selection of clearly defined—and where possible—mutually agreed goals.
3. Client becomes a willing and informed participant in his own therapy.
4. Constant evaluation of therapeutic interventions and their outcomes.

This process is comparable to the problem solving cycle in the nursing process; what it needs, we suggest, is a more socially attuned perspective than has previously been defined by behaviourists, namely, the framework of an interpersonally sensitive model of nursing.

The contribution of Hildegard Peplau (1952)

Behaviouristic approaches—when used exclusively as we earlier suggested—have a tendency to become mechanistic. The person can become lost in favour of his behaviour. To temper this process the philosophy of behaviourism needs to be combined with humane warmth; Peplau's concept of nursing comes to our aid here as it emphasises interpersonal awareness.

Peplau (1952) describes her approach as

a therapeutic activity, a healing art based on common goals between patients and nurses highlighting the need for mutual respect, growth and learning.

Health to Peplau is mediated by social awareness and sensitivity, it is a

> word symbol that implies forward movement of personality and on-going human processes in the direction of creative, constructive, productive, personal and community living.

Such concepts place the individuality of a client firmly back in the care picture.

More than any other model of nursing, Peplau's vision is tailored to a psychodynamic, interpersonal educative mode of care. The purpose of Peplau's model is to establish therapeutic exchange between the individual client and the nurse, who ideally needs to be

> . . . especially educated to recognise and respond to the need for help.

Dovetail the cognitive and structuring elements of behaviour therapy to the person sensitivity of this approach and a successful strategy emerges.

Peplau's 'philosophical approach' focuses upon the nature of the therapeutic relationship: its phases, which are described as growing out from an **orientation phase** (where the nurse is primarily concerned with the building of rapport) lead into a phase of **identification** (where the carer examines the client's unique state of need and response) to a further stage of **exploitation** (where the nurse acts as an educational agent—generating insights into feeling states and skills of self-care while building the client's self-worth and confidence) before the **resolution phase** of care (where nurse and client break their involvement and prepare for therapeutic independence, each from the other). The mutual dependence and interdependence of a nurse–patient relationship are clearly recognised in Peplau's approach.

Examine Figure 4.1 where Peplau's therapeutic relationship concept is teased out a little to illustrate its relevance to the nursing rôle. Though much has followed on from work done by others, Peplau's contribution is useful in orientating us to the social facilitation process that tends to thread its way through nursing models. It also goes some way to indicating just what we should be facilitating, namely:

— Health education and the reduction of anxiety.
— Understanding and meaning, so that our clients may better appreciate what is happening to them.
— The client's psycho-social energies towards therapeutic goals.
— Environmental stability, especially in regard to emotional cohesion and self-understanding.

A care example

The approach of a nurse therapist is qualitatively different from that of a nurse based within and responsible for, a clinical unit such as the ward. Nurse therapists work with a specific brief for each client referred, they are responsible for the overall management and movement of each client and decide on all aspects of care management following referral through to discharge to other workers. They also work from the premise that it is best to utilise existing personnel and clinical resources, in contrast to either taking over the client themselves or involving others alien to the client or his situation. Owing to their independent rôle, nurse therapists of necessity must keep careful records.

Clinical records in the following care example take three main forms:

1. Incident graphs tabulating the frequency of specific behaviour, a task performed by the resident clinical staff.
2. A care diary of involvement with the client, kept by the therapist.
3. A diary of feelings and responses, kept by the client.

Most of the data that follows is drawn from my own care diary. Though in the original account no headings existed, these have been added to orientate the reader to the various therapeutic phases and behavioural stages that arise.

Peplau's philosophy—throughout our subsequent narrative—serves as orientation to the therapeutic potential available within the

Fig. 4.1   An interpretive analysis of Peplau's model of care. Phases of the therapeutic relationship are given according to Peplau's model of interpersonal relationships

Phases	Characteristics/Relational dynamics	Nursing activities/Qualities
Orientation	Establishment of rapport and a therapeutic relationship along which understanding may flow to help the nurse appreciate the client's situation while the client and family gain insight into the dynamics of caring	Analyses: client's feelings; client's preconceptions and their own expectations; the rôle that personal attitudes play in nurse–patient relations.
Identification	Focuses upon the unique needs and reactions of the client; attempts to involve the client in self-care while resolving his feelings of helplessness	Identifies the nature of client response: participant interdependent with nurse; autonomous and independent from nurse; passive and dependent upon nurse
Exploitation	Helps client to explore his own feelings and responses while encouraging his self-sufficiency and confidence	Educates client to: his feelings and emotional reactions; activities of self-care; a sense of self-worth and trust
Resolution	A transition stage where the client is helped to terminate his involvement within the therapeutic relationship	Prepares client for: independent function; relinquishing of therapeutic support; discharge from care

nurse–client relationship; behaviour therapy here provides the frame for action; the latter therefore suggests *what* is to be done while the former *how* we may set about doing it.

Orientation/behaviour Stage 1 (summarised in Care Profile One)

Jim is now 42 years of age. Record review revealed that Jim had been in a large institution

---

CARE PROFILE No. 1

Name   Jim X   Behavioural stage   1

Date   Relationship phase   Orientation

Area   Hostel X

Care needs	Goals	Interventions	Outcomes
To assess Jim's potential and previous behaviour	To pool all information to date	Record review Team review	Jim is able to perform successfully in an environment he knows and trusts
To build up Jim's trust and acceptance of me so we may work together	For Jim to accept and use me as a resource	Daily visits Join Jim in his daily activities	Jim participates in games of draughts
		Share my reasons with Jim for taking an interest in him	Jim wishes to understand why he undresses and accepts my help

for mentally handicapped people since early childhood, following the death of his last surviving parent. He had grown up in the institution and by all accounts had 'fitted in well', working in the hospital canteen and presenting 'no problems to ward staff'. Jim was able to care for himself and was a prime candidate for transfer to the newly opened hostel in a nearby town when it opened. Since moving to the new hostel Jim had begun to behave strangely. The behaviour deemed problematic was Jim's recent habit of wandering around the hostel with no clothes on. Several of the other residents and their visitors had complained, but things were really brought to a head when a neighbour saw Jim wandering around the garden naked and called the police. Attempts to stop Jim undressing had proved to no avail. With the threat of discharge back to the parent institution hanging over him, referral was made to me as a nurse therapist serving the community.

The team review initiated care proper and all personnel involved with Jim met to discuss his previous behaviour pattern and to collate all recorded information. Hostel staff had recorded several incidents, variously classified as 'aggressive outbursts', 'attention-seeking behaviour', 'comfort behaviour' and 'depression'. Thus the hostel team had already indulged in behavioural diagnosis but without following a care strategy which would amend any of their diagnoses. In these early meetings with hostel staff I took the opportunity to share the philosophy of my approach, that is, the information of Figure 4.2 linking Peplau's therapeutic phases with the behavioural therapy stages to be addressed.

My next step was to meet Jim personally. I joined him in his hostel and as he made me tea, informed him of the reason for my visit, namely, that his undressing himself was causing embarrassment to those he lived with and that my job was to try and help him in whatever way possible. 'I'm alright' was his immediate response, shortly followed by 'I don't know what all the fuss is about'. I chose not to press the issue but rather enquired as to his hobbies and interests. Jim's hobbies were many; superficially, he appeared to be a well-adjusted middle-aged man of ami-

able disposition who looked older than his years and would readily be accepted in most communities. It seemed most appropriate to me to visit daily so that there could be a build-up of acceptance and trust, with a view to pursuing the subject of his undressing at a later more comfortable stage in our relationship. As my visits continued Jim began to appreciate me, initially, because I was able to play draughts with him in the late afternoon when he returned from work. He was a good player and mostly won with ease. I found myself liking him and feeling a little reluctant to proceed out from the social rôle circumstances had thrust upon me. Peplau makes mention of stereotypic responses and I was well aware of the danger of falling into the rôle of friend rather than therapist.

Identification/behaviour Stage 2 (summarised in Care Profile Two)

Our relationship gradually, and naturally, slipped into the Identification stage. Jim's response was primarily 'participant-independent' in character, here we seemed to be both clarifying each other's intent and checking out the reality of one another. Each week my observations were shared with other members of the care team and my intentions revised. My discussions with Jim from the third day onwards developed a therapeutic shape. Jim started to admit to 'not knowing what came over him' when he undressed himself. Though he was of higher ability than many of his hostel colleagues he was not able to self-reflect and analyse his own behaviour. One-to-one discussion with Jim led to a mutual decision to monitor events for a period of four weeks. The method of measurement would centre around Jim keeping a daily record of his thoughts, behaviour and feelings which I would help him with when I visited.

The above record, as was explained to Jim, would help us both to identify what led to his undressing. Jim also saw this as a means of improving his writing skills so that he could write off for all the bargains he saw in the Sunday papers. Jim in fact had set his mind on a pair of fleece-lined slippers. They were not found in

Fig. 4.2   Understanding the nature of the therapeutic relationship

Therapeutic phases of nurse–client relationship (? processes)	Behaviour aims/stages (? tasks)
Orientation Nurse and client meet as strangers, orientate to each other and establish rapport while working together to clarify and define the existing problem. Nurse notes personal reactions to client and seeks to avoid stereotypic responses that limit therapeutic potential; i.e. only doing tasks for the client, patronising him, parenting him so inducing dependence or ignoring the client's contribution	1. *Systematic measurement and assessment of presenting problems:* review of nursing records team discussion nursing diagnosis options recognised
Identification Client and nurse clarify each other's perception and expectations. Past experiences shading 'present meanings' examined, i.e. client's trust or mistrust of nursing staff, dependence upon or reactions against them etc. Client's selective response to nurse noted: participate interdependently; autonomous and independent; passive and dependent	2. *Selection and clarification of mutually agreed goals:* care plan goals assessed nursing interventions planned
Exploitation Client encouraged to take a responsible rôle in his own therapy, to explore his feelings, thoughts and responses, and to thus trust more in his own skills and resources. Nurse seeks to convey 'acceptance', 'concern' and 'trust' to enable this process. 'Wellness' becomes a goal in itself, nurse 'listens' and employs 'interpretive skills' to enable the client's understanding of all those 'avenues open' to him and 'agencies available' to help his self-adjustment	3. *Client to become a willing and informed participant in treatment:* periodic nurse–client reviews client sets his own goals nurse–client contact agreed adaptive behaviour reinforced
Resolution Termination of therapeutic relationship. Client encouraged to be less involved with helper. Nurse also establishes independence from the client. Client's needs are met regarding original problem, and other new goals orientated to enriching 'wellness' state may be reached, i.e. occupational and leisure interests	4. *Constant evaluation of therapeutic interventions:* long-term re-assessment planned ongoing support made available

local shops and he did not want others to write off for him, preferring to suddenly appear in them as a surprise. Independence was thus a feature and an asset of Jim's personality. By this stage Jim and I had developed a workable relationship where we each were able to accept the other; I could attune to his feelings by now without being preoccupied by my own need to demonstrate success or to over-control the outcomes of the interventions made.

Patience, being able to listen to the feelings of another and waiting comfortably in silence for an appropriate response were integral skills to therapy at this stage. Participant observation was the characteristic mode during this phase of the therapeutic process.

It was hoped that diary records would help to identify the time, place, number of clothes removed and causative factors prior to undressing behaviour. In order to produce an accurate record of the frequency of Jim's undressing behaviour and also a description of what took place when he did undress, assessment records were kept.

The first account recorded incidents of undressing within six-hourly periods, the second,

CARE PROFILE No. 2			
Name Jim X		Behavioural stage 2	
Date		Relationship phase Identification	
Area Hostel X			
Care needs	**Goals**	**Interventions**	**Outcomes**
To involve Jim in the identification of his own needs	For Jim to begin to re-cognise the pattern of his own behaviour	Helping Jim record his diary entries	Jim willingly records his thoughts and feelings
	For Jim to discuss the above and participate in forming future care goals	Encourage Jim to retain above record for 4 weeks	Jim participant-independent in his care relationship
		Shape conversation with Jim to encompass introspective reflection	Jim acknowledges be-wilderment as to why he undresses himself
			Jim wishes to find out why he keeps undressing him-self

the number of inappropriate undressing events. These were recorded by the nurse in charge, along with information about whether the incident was directly observed (and if so by whom) and if not who reported it, i.e. Jim, fellow patient, staff, visitor or other person.

A chart (Figure 4.3) was designed to be completed at the end of each shift by the nurse in charge. It was intended merely as a frequency count and included a trigger to complete the incident checklist (Figure 4.4).

Jim contracted to produce a detailed account of the behaviour occurring during each event. Additionally, he was asked to keep a daily diary of his thoughts and feelings about hostel life—who he spoke to and what he had done during the day.

Fig. 4.3 Frequency of undressing events. Nurse in charge to complete at end of each shift. √ = Yes, × = no.

Date	Did undressing occur?	Was it observed? If yes, by whom	If not observed who reported it?	Incident checklist completed?
25/10	√	Yes. S/N Jones	—	√
25/10	√	No.	resident	√
26/10	√	Yes. S/N Watson	—	√
26/10	√	No. —	resident	√
26/10	√	Yes. S/N Watson	—	√
27/10	√	Yes. S/N Watson	—	√
27/10	√	Yes. St/N Green	—	√
28/10	√	No. —	resident	√

Fig. 4.4   Incident analysis

Item	Date of clothes removal							
	25/10	25/10	26/10	26/10	26/10	26/10	27/10	28/10
Vest	✓	✓	✓	✓	✓			
Shirt	✓	✓	✓	✓	✓			
Jumper	✓	✓	✓	✓	✓			
Jacket	✓	✓	✓	✓	✓			
Pants	✓			✓	✓	✓	✓	✓
Trousers	✓			✓	✓	✓	✓	✓
Shoes & socks	✓			✓	✓	✓	✓	✓
Shoes only	✓			✓	✓	✓	✓	✓

It was explained that this would be private and Jim need not reveal its contents unless he wished.

Over a four-week period the reports showed a frequent occurrence of undressing behaviour— at least once a day. On each occasion a considerable amount of clothing was removed. It was decided to report this baseline information on two large graphs to be kept in the hostel office. Earlier records were continued to be kept and would be transferred to the graphs as soon as possible.

Review

When sufficient information was available from the above assessment strategies Jim's care was reviewed. This was done by addressing those questions we earlier identified in the Introduction to this chapter (Barker, 1982):

(1) What is the nature of the problems?
The baseline information gathered by care staff was transcribed into the following observable and measurable terms:

> 'Jim removes all or part of his clothing up to three times daily, between the hours of 9 am and 6 pm. He stays naked or partially dressed for periods of up to 30 minutes. During periods of nakedness he talks more often and more loudly than when clothed and in 50% of undressing events wanders from the hostel'.

(2) What should the final treatment goals be?
These were seen to stem from the above problem definition and reflect desirable outcomes for the client while replacing 'problem behaviour' with 'desirable behaviour'. Jim's goals were:

> not to remove any clothing between the hours of 9 am and 6 pm; to spend 1 hour in conversation with one other person daily.

(*Note*: Treatment goals are the end point of therapy, and as such may be modified or amended as treatment progresses.)

(3) When can treatment begin?
The care team agreed that therapeutic 'interventions', in the form of a designated programme could begin immediately.

(4) How should the programme be organised?
The care team agreed that a key worker for each duty period would carry out the programme for 30 minutes daily, with the nurse therapist deputising in their absence. The nurse therapist to co-ordinate feedback to other care staff.

(5) Which change techniques would be appropriate?
These are essential to clinical success; in Jim's case it was decided to utilise three different, though complementary activities. Firstly, a positive reinforcement approach based upon 'undressing-free time' being rewarded with conversation. Secondly, a two-tier 'rehearsal– alternative' behaviour model was used. This

sought to help Jim develop an awareness of the sorts of feelings and internal events which preceded his undressing, while equipping him with an alternative response to undressing. Thirdly, an elastic band—worn upon the wrist —was used as the cue signal; part of the key worker's activity was to practise feeling the way Jim did when he usually undressed.

(6) How should the programme be evaluated?
In Jim's case the original measures would be continued by care staff; in addition, they would record 'undressing-free periods' plus their own interventions. A reduction of undressing behaviour over a spell of two clear weeks would be perceived as a successful outcome. Follow-up measures would be given at one month, 6 months and 1 year periods, each of 2 weeks duration, to assess the long-term effects of the programme.

(7) Will the programme raise any ethical dilemmas?
The control of, or alteration of, an individual's behaviour, irrespective of their social, physical or psychological status presents care professionals with a dilemma. No behaviour programme can function effectively, nor ethically, without the proper consent of the individual it concerns (note the *Mental Health Act, Draft Code of Practice*, relating to the chapter on Consent to Treatment, 1983).

In addition, each individual is entitled to have an advocate of his choice involved in all discussions and decisions about therapy—this advocate should be someone outside the immediate care environment, e.g. friend, relative, etc. These issues need to be addressed and discussed within the care setting, and openly agreed upon by carers and client alike. In Jim's case, Jim himself was deemed to be of a degree of ability where he could personally be involved; he as client consented to the programme suggested and understood that he could halt it when and if he desired.

Exploitation/behaviour Stage 3 (summarised in Care Profile Three)

After the four-week observation period, a four-week treatment phase was initiated involving a

variety of behavioural approaches. The first involved positive reinforcement, a technique which rewards appropriate behaviour with previously identified reinforcers (see Barker 1982, Chapters 7 and 8 for a more detailed discussion).

It was established after consultation with Jim that the principal reinforcer would be social interaction with nurses. For every hour that he went without undressing he would get ten minutes conversation with a nurse of his choice. Again, there was a requirement that accurate records be kept of the reinforcement schedule (see Figure 4.5). This initially high rate of reinforcement is important when establishing new behaviour; the frequency of reinforcement can be lengthened and the required appropriate behaviour increased at a later date. Secondly, a direct approach was also made to inhibit undressing behaviour when it began. To this end, Jim was given an elastic band to place on his wrists; whenever he thought of undressing or began to undress he was to snap the band lightly on his wrist and immediately engage someone in a conversation for approximately five minutes. This technique is based upon the premise that behaviour is determined by those activities which preceded plus those consequences that follow, i.e.:

Antecedents→Behaviour→Consequences

It provides opportunities for the client to opt out of his continuing chain of behaviour. Thirdly, undressing behaviour was rehearsed via rôle-play.

Much rehearsal was needed with Jim to identify the particular thoughts and feelings that preceded his undressing. He identified 'loneliness' and 'depression' as the main emotions present when he undressed. The key nurse in charge of the programme rehearsed several times the sequence of events, asking Jim to imagine feeling lonely, encouraging him to think about undressing, and to remove a piece of clothing. As he began to do this Jim was instructed to snap his elastic band and seek someone out for conversation.

This rehearsal identified three stages for Jim. Firstly, feelings of loneliness and depression;

secondly, getting into the right environment—which to him was a public place where he could be observed, and thirdly, the taking-off of pieces of clothing in order to gain attention from others. Again this needed to be recorded. Jim was asked to record for himself when he used his band and how often. Figure 4.6 shows Jim's diary of events.

After four weeks, Jim's behaviour was reduced considerably as we can see from graphs of Figures 4.7 and 4.8. The actual occurrence of undressing had decreased from about twice daily

CARE PROFILE No. 3			

Name	Jim X	Behavioural stage	3
Date		Relationship phase	Exploitation
Area	Hostel X		

Care needs	Goals	Interventions	Outcomes
To systematically record Jim's behaviour and those changes that occur within it	To identify the time, place, number of clothes removed and causative factors involved in Jim's undressing behaviour	Participant observation Care diary of day-to-day conversation and interventions with Jim Four-hourly recording of Jim's inappropriate undressing behaviour by nurse in charge on frequency chart (Fig. 4.3) Incident checklist commenced (Fig. 4.4) Jim contracted to describe his undressing behaviour in his diary	Records and relationship reinforced simultaneously. Loneliness appears to be a factor Baseline behaviour established over recording 4-week period Jim identifies loneliness as a precipitating factor in his undressing behaviour
To use Jim's own requested reward to reinforce his retention of dress	To reinforce positive behavioural responses	Jim to get 10 minutes with nurse of his choice for every hour of remaining fully clothed To record periods of social reinforcement (see Fig. 4.5.)	Jim's undressing has diminished sharply Jim's need for social reinforcement gradually diminishing with regard to nurse contact (week 2)
For Jim to control his own behaviour	To inhibit negative behavioural responses	Jim to snap an elastic band on his wrist and engage in a five minutes conversation when he feels the need to undress	Jim says he finds it easier to initiate conversation (week 2)

CARE NEEDS	GOALS	INTERVENTIONS	OUTCOMES
To reinforce Jim's insight into his own behaviour	For Jim to examine those emotions which attend his undressing	Rehearsal of undressing behaviour Charge Nurse will perform above with behaviour therapist and in his absence	Loneliness and depression identified by Jim as present prior to his undressing Jim recognises his need to find an audience for his undressing Jim has come to realise he only undresses to gain attention from others Jim's undressing has further diminished to less than once a week (2nd week of programme) Jim says he feels less lonely (3rd week of programme)

to less than once a week; the event itself had been reduced to the removal of one or two items of clothing only. As a consequence of the care plan promoting conversation with people, Jim spent less time alone and openly stated that he felt less lonely.

Resolution/behaviour Stage 4 (summarised in Care Profile Four)

Long-term re-assessment dates were fixed at those periods previously identified, i.e. 6 months and one year. Care staff programmed time periods into their diaries and I arranged to return to the clinical area for one day in each of the two-week periods when re-assessment was occurring. Key workers were seen as providing the ongoing support to Jim; they were also to monitor the possibility of relapse.

Resolution of the therapeutic relationship I had enjoyed with Jim had already started to occur as key workers were introduced into the programme. I agreed in discussion with Jim to return and see him again, setting a date to meet

him following work in one month, and three months following that. I also gave him my workbase phone number so that he might leave a message for me to contact him before then, should he feel the necessity.

The above were drawn up in Care Profile 4 to orientate the care staff to future evaluation while framing the direction of assessment in our next meeting. As care was ongoing and outcomes were in the future, this latter column was left blank.

Conclusion

We have attempted in this care study to share some of the effect that results from dovetailing behaviour therapy to the psychodynamic approach of Hildegard Peplau. We have endeavoured to keep the perspective of care simplistic, but attuned to the interpersonal and therapeutic dynamics that permeate nursing action.

We have further attempted to illustrate that:

It is likely that the nursing process is educative and therapeutic when nurse and patient can come to

Fig. 4.5   Reinforced schedule—completed hourly

√ = Yes, × = No

Date	Time	Event free?		If 'yes' please sign after 10 minutes' comments
1/11	10.00	√		M. Brown
	11.00		×	M. Brown
	12.00	√		M. Brown
	13.00	√		M. Brown
	14.00		×	M. Brown
	15.00		×	M. Brown
	16.00	√		M. Brown
	17.00	√		M. Brown
	18.00	√		M. Brown
2/11	10.00	√		M. Brown
	11.00	√		M. Brown
	12.00	√		M. Brown
	13.00		×	M. Brown
	14.00	√		M. Brown
	15.00	√		J. Quinn
	16.00	√		J. Quinn
	17.00	√		J. Quinn
	18.00	√		J. Quinn
3/11	10.00		×	J. Quinn
	11.00	√		J. Quinn
	12.00	√		J. Quinn
	13.00	√		J. Quinn
	14.00	√		C. Devonish
	15.00	√		C. Devonish
	16.00	√		C. Devonish
	17.00	√		C. Devonish
	18.00	√		C. Devonish
4/11	10.00	√		M. Brown
	11.00	√		M. Brown
	12.00	√		M. Brown
	13.00	√		M. Brown
	14.00	√		M. Brown
	15.00	√		J. Quinn
	16.00	√		J. Quinn
	17.00	√		J. Quinn
	18.00	√		J. Quinn

Fig. 4.6. Times I wanted to undress

Date . . . .

Day	Time	How I felt	What I did
Monday	7 pm	Tired, bored, no one to talk to	Spoke to Joe
Thursday	9 am	Didn't want to go to work	Talked to Joe, he went with me to work
Friday	3 pm	Felt lonely	Told Anne I felt lonely, went for a walk with her
Saturday	6 pm	Felt bored	Took off my shirt and shoes and walked in garden
Sunday	3 pm	Wanted visitors like Fred; no one came to see me	Told Joe I wanted to undress

Fig. 4.7 Frequency graph

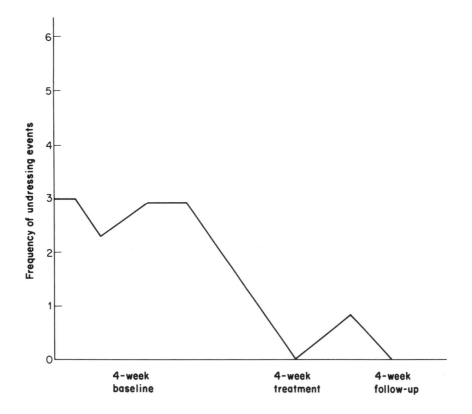

Fig. 4.8   Incident analysis graph

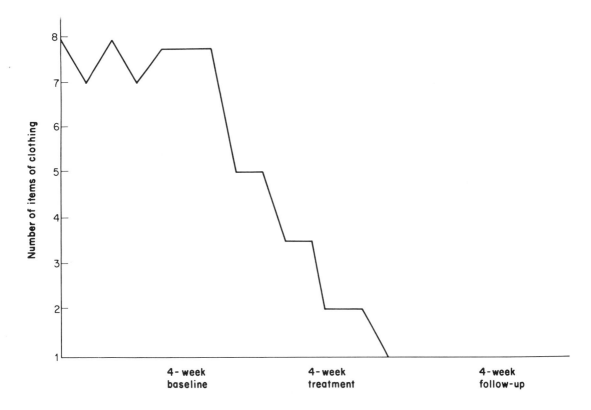

know and to respect each other, as persons who are alike, and yet different, as persons who share in the solution of problems.

(Peplau, 1952)

Ultimately, the success of this chapter depends on how well we have conveyed the necessity to combine social sensitivity with rigorously assessed goal-planning while breathing life into the rôle of the nurse as an educational catalyst:

> When the serial and goal-directed nature of the nursing process is appreciated, nursing plans can be designed to include the steps necessary to make illness an eventful experience in learning for patients. Understanding of the meaning of the experience to the patient is required in order for nursing to function as an educative, therapeutic, maturing force.

(Peplau, 1952)

If readers are caused to reflect upon their own therapeutic potential and to more confidently combine the rôle of friend with that of carer, this chapter will have been deemed successful by its authors.

Critique

Behaviourism, which focuses upon the external responses of an individual and seeks to explore ways of modifying their 'behavioural show', seems far removed from the rationale of Peplau's model of 'therapeutic phases'. Too much may have been attempted in the chapter; is it really productive to reconcile two such distinctly different perspectives?

In mitigation, it must be recognised that Peplau's work is primarily focused upon the psychiatric nursing rôle, and so would seem a suitable vehicle to re-educate a psychiatrically disturbed client, such as Jim; but is this 'mental illness' orientation generally relevant to the field of mental handicap?

CARE PROFILE No. 4

Name	Jim X		Behavioural stage	4
Date			Relationship phase	Resolution
Area	Hostel X			

Care needs	Goals	Interventions	Outcomes
To provide long-term re-evaluation	Identify times, venue, periods for this to occur	Nurse therapist to visit Jim in between times to assess his progress	
	To identify carers who will monitor Jim's activities	Key workers to monitor everyday events	
		Records of undressing and treatment inputs to be retained for six months	
For Jim to feel an access route is available to nurse therapist should he desire it	For Jim to initiate contact should he feel it necessary	Base phone number given to Jim	

Peplau defines nursing as '. . . a maturing force and educative instrument' (Peplau, 1952); maturation and education are highly desirable nursing intentions applicable to the care of persons with mental handicap.

Behaviour modification in mental handicap has all too often been mechanistically applied, forcing conformity rather than liberating skills or awareness. Perhaps this is somewhat redressed by the emphasis of this work, if not, then it fails, for the thrust of this chapter is founded upon the premise that interpersonal skills are the most effective techniques for behavioural shaping, and self-learning the most appropriate goal of care.

Paul Barber

Salient questions

1. Has the chapter convincingly redressed the mechanistic tendency of behaviour modification?
2. Is Peplau's model of care well served by 'marriage' to behaviourism?
3. Are the two approaches chosen at variance with each other?
4. Does the care study illuminate a unique and useful approach to care or just confuse perspectives which are clearer—and more effective—when used alone?
5. Is the format of care suited to mentally handicapped clients?

References

Bandura AL 1977 *Social Learning Theory*, Prentice-Hall, New Jersey.

Barker PJ 1982 *Behaviour Therapy Nursing*, Croom Helm, London.

Barker PJ 1985 *Patient Assessment in Psychiatric Nursing*, Croom Helm, London.

Beck AT 1976 *Cognitive Therapy and Emotional Disorders*, International Universities Press, New York.

Child D 1981 *Psychology and the Teacher* (3rd edition), Holt, Rinehart & Winston, London.

Ellis A 1962 *Reason and Emotion in Psychotherapy*, Stuart, New York.

Griffiths P 1985 The treatment of bathing and eating problems in a mentally handicapped woman. In: PJ Baker & D Fraser (eds), *The Nurse as Therapist*, Croom Helm, London.

Harkin W 1985 The management of chronic pain. In: PJ Baker & D Fraser (eds), *The Nurse as Therapist*, Croom Helm, London.

Kazdim AE & Wilson GT 1978 *Evaluation of Behavior Therapy: Issues, Evidence and Research Strategies*, Ballinger, Cambridge, Mass.

McFall RM 1976 Behavioral training: A skill-acquisition approach to clinical problems. In: JT Spence, RC Carson & JW Thitaut (eds), *Behavioural Approaches to Therapy*, General Learning Press, New Jersey.

McPherson FM, Barker P, Hunter M & Fraser D 1978 A course in behaviour modifications, *Nursing Times* (20th July).

Mahoney MJ 1974 *Cognition and Behavior Modification*, Ballinger, Cambridge, Mass.

Marks IM, Hallam RS, Connolly J & Philpott R 1977 *Nursing in Behavioural Psychotherapy*, Royal College of Nursing, London.

Meichenbaum DH 1975 *Cognitive Behavior Modification*, Plenum Press, New York.

Peplau H 1952 *Interpersonal Relations in Nursing: A Conceptual Frame of Reference for Psychodynamic Nursing*, Putnam & Sons, New York.

Stevanson L 1974 *Seven Theories of Human Nature*, Oxford University Press, Oxford & New York, quoting from BF Skinner, *Verbal Behaviour* (1957).

Watson JB 1924 *Behaviourism* (revised edition, 1930), p. 104; quoted in L Stevanson, *Seven Theories of Human Nature*, Oxford University Press, Oxford & New York (1974).

5

A process approach to ward management: replacing routines with nursing models— a managerial perspective

Margaret Williams

Summary

A novel concept introduced by the author is that of applying models of nursing—which were primarily intended for use with the individual—to the larger scale of ward management. Comparison is drawn between ward care fifteen years ago and that of the present day—little is seen to have changed. The chapter argues that routines must first be changed before care can improve, for these frustrate gains which can accrue from the use of nursing models.

The philosophy of the General Nursing Council for England and Wales 1982 Syllabus of Training is examined, along with other progressive doctrines.

Orem's 'self-care' model is specifically chosen to provide a rationale of clinical management, critical analysis of care being made via this vehicle. Resident training is explored in the light of the above analysis and a person-centred style of management proposed to remedy unproductive traditional practices.

Roper's model of nursing is further employed to think through managerial strategy· and isolate problems.

Periodically, insights which have arisen from personal practice are shared, to convey a feeling of first-hand managerial experience. The viewpoint contrasts sharply with the more academic orient-ation of nurse educators, and the 'care-plan' approach of clinical practitioners.

Paul Barber

Introduction

This chapter examines the work of two authors, Orem (1980) and Roper *et al.* (1983), and describes how the application of these models may help nursing staff to examine their own work patterns, with a view to changing from 'routine orientation' to modes of 'client-centredness'. This not only affects ward organisation, bene-fiting residents, but may also provide nursing staff with greater job satisfaction.

Daily life on the ward in a hospital for the mentally handicapped resident often revolves around basic routines: dressing, eating, toileting and washing; a weekly film show, occasional outings, and short periods of occupational therapy to punctuate this pattern. Otherwise, residents and staff talk, play, or just sit on the ward or in the outside 'airing courts'. To the nurse, routine life on the ward corresponds to the abilities of their clients; to move away from these routines is seen to require a development in the behaviour range of such clients: moreover, to abandon routines before such developments is seen as endangering the balance of the whole group—with the consequence that conservation and excessive safety measures may be a com-moner feature than innovation.

The following description of ward life comes from the 1960s and concerns an area where clients were deemed to be 'severely subnormal':

'Severe subnormality' referred to those residents who were highly dependent on the ward staff, most being unable to speak and needing help with all aspects of their daily life. The ward in question had 35 male residents between the ages of 19 and 45. It was usually staffed in the day by two qualified staff, two unqualified nursing staff, and two or three staff on a part time basis.

The ward 'then'

The nurse in charge spent a good deal of the morning in the office making 'arrangements' and 'communicating' with the Central Nursing Office. The major pivots of daily life were the meal times, for example, the midday meal. At 11.30 am every day, the most senior nurses on duty organised the necessary arrangements.

As midday approached tables were laid for dinner, usually by a resident—from another ward. The necessary number of plates and dishes were put ready near the serving hatch. The food arrived in a heated trolley from the central hospital kitchen. Serving began. The residents' involvement in preparing for dinner was non-existent. The majority were not seen as capable of helping.

The nurse in charge of serving announced that dinner was now ready. This announcement, in the day room, got an immediate response from residents. They began moving out into the dining room. There was no need to provide much direction, nurses ensured that no one was left behind, either in the day room or in the toilets. Dinner was soon under way. Residents sat at tables laid for six. The nurses divided residents into familiar groups, a strategy found by experience to minimise feeding difficulties. One resident who persistently 'stole' food from others was fed quickly and then locked outside the dining room. On entering the corridor he stood, nose to glass, quietly staring through the window of the door back into the dining room. He rarely wandered off, waiting and hoping that he would be let back in. Of the 35 residents, nine were spoon-fed by the nurses on duty and the resident helper, and the rest either ate with their spoons or hands. Nurses were kept busy providing the

food, attempting to keep all diners at the table, and holding down the level of noise.

Then, difficulties at meal times were minimised by the hard work of the available staff. Without radical reorganisation, attempts to help clients with their table skills was an uphill job, if not an impossibility. One nurse spent months trying to teach a resident how to eat with a spoon, but after a week's holiday he went back to square one. This did not surprise the nurse, but confirmed the idea that 'programmes' were largely not worth it. The formula—that severe subnormality meant lack of basic social skills, which meant an inability to eat properly—provided a workable definition of behaviour at meal times. The nurse attempted to reconcile authoritative ideas about subnormality with her practical experience on the ward. The nurse also saw her rôle as being both custodian and guardian of those rejected from society.

The ward 'now'

I know this ward well, I worked there! And today? Is it a great deal different? The number of residents on the ward has been reduced to twenty and the environment and ward furniture are much brighter; there are many more occupational therapists employed in the hospital and fifteen of the residents attend the occupational therapy department, thus allowing the ward staff much more time to do activities and training programmes with the remaining residents; but, what in fact happens? After fifteen residents have departed for the occupational therapy department and the ward staff have had third cup of tea—what next? The Charge Nurse goes to the ward office and 'does' his paper work, the Youth Opportunity person polishes the office furniture (despite the fact that there is a ward domestic); two nursing auxiliaries put the laundry away— and the residents? A nursing auxiliary sits with one eye on them and with the other on the TV.

Residents no longer come from other wards to help with odd jobs, so as lunch-time approaches a nursing auxiliary lays the dining-room tables and puts the plates and dishes ready for the arrival of the heated food trolley from the central hospital kitchen.

The residents arrive back from the occupational therapy department and the nurse in charge serves up the meal; the staff hand the meals around and feed the residents who are unable to feed themselves. Time is pressing—after all—the residents have to get back to the occupational therapy department on time.

Social institutions are subject to a certain inertia. Once set up they tend to be self-perpetuating and resistant to change; updating and appraisal must occur continuously to counter such apathy.

The Nodder Report (1977) gave indications of how standards of care might be improved and changes be introduced into hospitals for both the mentally ill and the mentally handicapped. The report recommended that there should be clearly written operational policies at district, hospital and ward level, and that each operational policy should describe (i) the goals of the service for its residents, and, (ii) the means by which these goals were to be attained.

Guidelines were given for planning the daily pattern of clients' lives so that all residents, however severely disturbed or handicapped, are given an opportunity to participate as much as possible in normal daily activities. The report goes on to say that

> all patients are in hospital to receive help for their individual problem and it is important, therefore, that there is a clearly defined individual programme of care for each patient

and,

> Each patient should receive treatment, therapy, education or training specifically designed to solve his individual problems and reviewed on a regular basis.

To achieve this

> A clearly written programme plan should be prepared for each patient specifying the individual goals for that patient and the method to attain each goal.

These concepts suggest the way forward for positive management attitudes and the planning of nursing care to suit individual client needs. Leading from this, there is a requirement for a framework around which to base individual nursing-care programmes—and that means nursing models.

Reflection upon 'change'

The 1982 Syllabus of Training provides a good baseline for qualified nurses to understand their rôle and develop strategies that bring about change. Quoting from the introduction, the syllabus states that

> The function of the nurse for people with mental handicap is directly and skillfully to assist the individual and his family, whatever the handicap, in the acquisition, development and maintenance of those skills that, given the necessary ability, would be performed unaided, and to do this in such a way as to enable independence to be gained as rapidly and fully as possible in an environment that maintains a quality of life that would be acceptable to fellow citizens of the same age.
>
> (Adapted from Henderson, 1966)

The philosophy of the syllabus is based on three principles: first, that people with mental handicap have the same rights and as far as possible the same responsibilities as other members of the community; second, that they have the right to live like others in the community and to receive services that meet their changing needs; thirdly, that they should receive additional help from professional services to allow full recognition and expression of their individuality.

> These principles will only be achieved if the nurse has the skills and ability to participate in multi-disciplinary team work in its fullest skill sharing sense.
>
> (*ibid.*)

Nurses too often are embroiled in the practical routines of the ward, which in turn become 'the routines' they live by. They rush to get through their task-orientated duties and forget the individual needs of their clients. For example, all of the residents must be bathed before breakfast, all must be dressed by 9 am so that the staff may then be free to do the other ward routines of putting the laundry away and making the beds before lunch time!

Significant work on the practice of care for the mentally handicapped has been carried out by groups from the Institute of Education, London (King and Raynes, 1968; Raynes and King, 1968; King, Raynes and Tizard, 1971; Tizard, 1968). These studies identified four interrelated characteristics of the hospitalised care: **rigidity, block treatment, depersonalisation,** and **social distance**.

(1) Rigidity
This was the most commonly presented feature; the routine of the ward was often such that the same practices were carried out at the same time on the same days.

(2) Block treatment
Residents being managed as a group rather than as individuals.

(3) Depersonalisation
Very little evidence was found of any opportunities for privacy or expression of individuality.

(4) Social distance between staff and patients
Interaction between staff and residents was limited to basic functional necessities with very few attempts at personal relationships.

When nurses put their ward before their clients the above features predominate; but what are the alternatives? Henderson in 1966 gave us her definition of nursing as follows:

> The unique function of the nurse is to assist the individual, sick or well, in the performance of those activities contributing to health or its recovery (or to a peaceful death) that he would perform unaided if he had the necessary strength, will or knowledge, and to do this in such a way as to help him gain independence as rapidly as possible.

By helping the client to gain independence through the use of the 'nursing process' an 'individual' approach is achieved in contrast to a 'task-orientated' care pattern where instrumental activities dominate.

Sundeen *et al.* (1976) expanded this further via the concept of nursing as a 'client-orientated profession' that effects changes in the clients' bio-psychological environment to promote health, learning and growth; and noted particularly, that the nurse 'engages the client as the partner in health care'.

Mayers (1972) proposes that to achieve nursing's purpose, a nurse needs a philosophy and an operational model. A model is defined by Riehl and Roy (1980) as

> a symbolic depiction in logical terms of an idealised system . . . , a conceptual model of reality. It shows the features of a discipline and gives direction to a cluster of laws that are selected to form a theoretical system.

'Theory', is then defined as 'the workings inside the model'. Both 'theory' and 'model' provide separate conceptions of reality for their own purposes—the theory emphasising, explaining and predicting a certain empirical reality, and the model showing the parts of nursing and how they are related.

Nursing models have developed logically in an attempt to make better sense of what nurses do and should do, and seek to bond such insights creatively to the delivery of care. Such insights tend to focus upon:

(a) The condition of the individual recipient of care.
(b) The causation of those problems which are likely to require nursing interventions.
(c) An assessment process to address the above.
(d) A framework for planning and goal-setting.
(e) A philosophy regarding the purposes, direction and quality of nursing interventions during implementation of a nursing care plan.
(f) A means of evaluating the quality and effects of the care given.

All of these strike at the heart of 'ward routines'—they are the cure for inertia.

Orem's self-care model

Orem describes self-care as 'an adult's personal contribution to his own health and well being'. This concept is applicable to the health of individuals rather than to their state of ill health and is organised around individual activities which maintain health. It is a model which values individual responsibilities and argues for prevention and health education as key aspects of nursing intervention. Orem sees nurses as being concerned with the individual's need and ability to perform self care to sustain health, to recover from disease or injury, or to cope with the effects of disease or injury.

The majority of the people who reside in hospitals for the mentally handicapped are not physically ill; many are physically able people who, given the opportunity, could contribute to their own well-being. All too frequently this fundamental right is denied them by the nurse who automatically performs care action for them. Doing things 'for' our clients may be seen as caring for them, but doing things 'with' them is nearer to therapy.

Orem's model portrays individuals as functional integrated wholes with strong motivational urges to achieve self care. Clients here are viewed as active agents who contribute to their own care programme. The rôle of the nurse is one of facilitating clients in the direction of self-care capabilities, capabilities which may be frustrated by the institutional constraints of ward life. We noted in our earlier account how residents may be denied the opportunity of learning to feed themselves because it was seen to be easier and quicker by nurses to do this task themselves. Such 'block regimes' de-skill clients. 'Doing' things for clients is only one of the ways, identified by Orem, by which nurses may meet care goals, i.e.

—Doing or acting for another
—Guiding or directing another
—Providing physical support
—Providing psychological support
—Providing an environment which enables development
—Teaching another

The above suggest that care is more a feature of enabling others to help themselves than rushing into routines that do things for them.

When using Orem's model as a basis for the planning and implementation of care and training for mentally handicapped people, the nurse must be aware of the 'balance' between the client's ability 'to act' to achieve self care, and the 'demands' their environment makes upon them. Ward environments must be tailored to meet client needs, not the other way round. Orem suggests that there are six universal self-care needs; the need for:

1. Sufficient intake of air, water, nutrition
2. Satisfactory eliminative functions
3. Activity balanced with rest
4. Time spent alone balanced with time spent with others
5. Prevention of danger to self
6. Being 'normal'

A healthy individual has sufficient self-care ability to meet these functions. Nursing interventions are required only when an individual is unable to achieve and maintain a balance between their self-care abilities and present environmental demands. Such a situation occurs when self-care demands exceed self-care abilities. Opportunities must be planned where handicapped residents can learn self-care skills. But before nurses attempt this, they must first evaluate the ward. Figure 5.1 demonstrates the use of Orem's model in ward evaluation. The universal care aims are listed, and these, when applied to the ward in question, are contrasted against those changes to ward routines necessary to train residents to self care.

Addressing the ward environment before commencing individual care planning is possibly the best way to build up a solid care foundation, otherwise, individual programmes can be disturbed by unsympathetic ward routines.

But before change is attempted, certain relationships need to be recognised.

(i) There is a need to assess those demands being made on the individual for self care, and to assess

Fig. 5.1   Using Orem's model to evaluate the ward: thinking through ward routines

Care aims	Changes to ward routines necessary to improve on these
Sufficient intake of air, water, nutrition At present no opportunity for residents to help themselves to cold drinks when they feel a need, though all have the potential to do so	Need to teach the resident group skills in the preparation of cold drinks and allow access to kitchen during periods when domestic activity is conducive to do so Brief domestic staff and night staff regarding this proposal
Satisfactory eliminative functions Not sufficient privacy in toilet areas. No locks on inside of cubicles	Place simple locks on inside of toilet doors with colour coding or engaged mechanism observable from without
Activity balanced with rest Residents appear reluctant to go out without nurse and walk in hospital grounds	Discuss possible reasons for this with ward staff Establish that residents know the choices open to them with regard to 'freedom of movement'
Time spent alone balanced with time spent with others Not sufficient privacy available, should a client demand it, within the ward	Could TV be placed in an area other than the main day room? Discuss options open to us with fellow staff during handover Would the Friends Association be prepared to raise money for a library reading room next to the existing library? Talk with senior managers regarding this
Prevention of danger to the self Check the level of staff awareness regarding fire drill	Check that clients are aware of danger areas and emergency procedures See that all staff are familiar with fire drill and have been on a fire-prevention course in the past year
Being normal Staff don't appear conversant with the philosophy of 'normalisation'	Set up ward based tutorials to improve awareness here Check the best area for staff to visit to see this in operation Have a word with the School of Nursing and In-Service Training areas to see what help they may suggest in this venture

the individual's ability to meet these demands. These two processes form the first stage of an assessment procedure from which decisions can be made regarding the need for nursing intervention.

(ii) If a self-care deficit is identified as existing, a nurse must establish the reasons for it. In the care of the mentally handicapped a deficit may exist because he/she does not possess sufficient knowledge to respond to self-care demands, or he/she may have insufficient skill to carry out the self-care activities.

(iii) The deficit of a self-care activity could be due to the lack of privacy in the ward, the lack of opportunity to take risks or just the absence of 'normal' environmental stimulation. The nurse must then assess whether the resident is able to engage in self care and finally assess their potential for re-establishing, or in the case of the mentally handicapped, establishing such care in the future.

(iv) During the process of planning and goal-setting, the nurse must keep objectives patient-centred. Orem emphasises the need for the nurse to negotiate with the patient at the planning stage whether nursing intervention is to be wholly compensatory, partly compensatory or educative/developmental.

Leading on from the identification of changes to ward routines necessary to improve individual self-care aims (as outlined in Figure 5.1), the six universal self-care needs suggested by Orem's model can be used as a basis for the planning and implementation of care. By using Orem's principles nurses may employ a goal-setting approach as an essential part of problem solving, thus providing direction to care, rationale to specific actions, and the setting of observable and measurable goals. All this makes evaluation of training programmes feasible.

Set out in Figure 5.2 are examples of training programmes related to our earlier findings (Figure 5.1). This list is by no means exhaustive, and is only representative of the multitude of programmes available using Orem's self-care model.

By addressing those questions presented by Orem's work (Figure 5.2) a philosophy for the ward may be defined, that is to say, a rationale or conceptual framework may arise from your clinical enquiry and force appraisal of such as:

What is the overall purpose of this unit?
How do we seek to achieve its purpose?
Who dictates the 'tone' and 'shape' of the ward's culture? Its clients, the nurses who staff it, the management policy, medical staff or tradition?

What is done well here and what do we fail to do?
Who cares for the staff and how do we support each other?
Do we support an educational, medical, psychological, or nursing model of care within our clinical area?
Are we actively therapeutic or just 'hotelier' in our service?

In applying Orem's self-care model, the nurse should bear in mind Yura and Walsh's (1978) remarks that

> Nursing is an encounter with a client (and his family) in which the nurse observes, supports, communicates, ministers and teaches, she contributes to the maintenance of optimum health and provides care during illness until the client is able to assume responsibility for the fulfillment of their own basic needs.

Some nurses in mental handicap view Orem's self-care model as limited and inappropriate to their work; their clients, they argue, do not have the physical, sensory or intellectual ability to achieve self care. Possibly Orem's model works best in ward environments where the less profoundly handicapped person resides; if this is so, another model of care is necessary for our less fortunate clients; the work of Roper *et al.* (1983) may be usefully employed here.

Roper's activities of living model

This model focuses upon twelve activities of living:

(i) Maintaining a safe environment
The nurse herself will need to assess whether she is maintaining a safe environment for her clients, while at the same time allowing the space and flexibility for them to take risks and grow personally and socially.

(ii) Communication
At what level is the person capable of communicating, what does he communicate and which

Fig. 5.2 Using Orem's model to develop resident training programmes

Identified problem related to self-care aim	Aim to be achieved	Means by which aim is to be achieved	Method to assist achievement of objectives	Assistance necessary from other staff
Sufficient intake of air, water, nutrition				
Residents are not used to helping themselves to cold drinks from the kitchen at appropriate times	Each resident to learn how to prepare cold drinks	Teach each resident how to: (i) measure out the correct amount of squash for one portion; (ii) serve drinks to fellow residents during mid-morning/afternoon periods; (iii) wash, dry and put away cups after each use	Allow resident access to the kitchen during mid-morning/afternoon, evening and night time	Supervision by day and night nursing staff, ward O.T. staff Supervision by ward O.T. staff, domestic staff, day and night nursing staff
Satisfactory eliminative functions				
Residents are not used to locking toilet doors, so even on trips outside of the hospital, toilet doors are left open causing embarrassment to other people	Each resident to learn to lock the toilet door whilst in use	Teach each resident how to: (i) identify if a toilet door is locked/unlocked; (ii) lock the toilet door when in use; (iii) unlock the toilet door after use	Training programmes inside and outside of the hospital token economy systems	Day and night nursing staff, ward O.T. staff to support this programme

Fig. 5.2 (continued)

Identified problem related to self-care aim	Aim to be achieved	Means by which aim is to be achieved	Method to assist achievement of objectives	Assistance necessary from other staff
Activity balanced with rest Residents appear reluctant to go without nurse and walk in the hospital grounds	Each resident to take a certain amount of exercise each day, independently of nursing staff	For each resident: (i) identify likes/dislikes for leisure activities; (ii) ensure that they know of all leisure activities which are taking place in the hospital; (iii) encouragement to attend leisure activities of their choice; (iv) give a specific errand to run each day; (v) encouragement to visit friends on other wards	Individual assessment Information board Staff Talks Token economy system	Familiarise following: All nursing staff, ward O.T. staff, recreation officer All staff All staff Staff on other wards
Time spent alone balanced with time spent with others Residents are used to sitting in the ward dayroom only for all indoor activities, i.e. watching TV, talking, sewing, knitting, reading, writing. Therefore there is no opportunity for privacy	Each resident to be given the opportunity to be alone when necessary for activities such as reading, writing, listening to their own radio	Each resident to be taught the different ward areas that they can use for their individual activities e.g. quiet room, own bedroom	Staff training to encourage residents to use appropriate ward areas	All staff Ward O.T. staff
Prevention of danger to self Residents do not always respond appropriately to fire-drill exercises, because often they are told in advance that they are happening	Every resident to respond appropriately to the ringing of the fire bell	Teach each resident: (i) action to be taken upon the ringing of the fire bell; (ii) correct exit to take; (iii) correct assembly point; (iv) how to behave at the assembly point	Staff-training: arrange mock fire drills to be held at different times. Residents and other staff not to be informed of mock fire drills	Fire officer Maintenance or other appropriate department

Fig. 5.2 (continued)

Identified problem related to self-care aim	Aim to be achieved	Means by which aim is to be achieved	Method to assist achievement of objectives	Assistance necessary from other staff
Being normal Residents are institutionalised and routines are such that they receive block treatment as opposed to individualised care	Each resident as an individual, is given the opportunity to exercise choice over daily living activities	Each resident should have the opportunity to: (i) go to bed (within reason) at a time of their own choice; (ii) have a 'lie in' at the weekends or when they are not working; (iii) have a choice of menu; (iv) with help initially, choose and buy their own clothes; (v) choose their own hairstyle; (vi) be consulted as to where they would like to go on holiday; (vii) be consulted on appropriate self-care training programmes etc.	Staff training day and night on re-education of attitudes Give access to fashion catalogues Taking on shopping trips Give access to hair-styling books Give access to travel brochures Following assessment, discuss programmes with residents	Night staff Catering department Hairdresser Para-medical staff, as appropriate

method of communication best suits him? If he is immobile which is the position in which to place him so that others can communicate to him and he can communicate to others, even if it is only through eye contact? This is an area of need where the nurse should seek the assistance of the speech therapist, who can not only assist in the assessment and planning stage but can also help to carry programmes out. Nursing staff can also receive the necessary training from the speech therapist in order to develop their skills in this area to the benefit of the patients.

(iii) Breathing
Any physical abnormality which may interfere with breathing needs to be noted so that advice can be sought from the physiotherapist as to the most advantageous positioning to use.

(iv) Eating and drinking
Assessment will be required of the patient's capabilities and disabilities. The nurse will need to know (in addition to knowing how capable he is of feeding himself) the types of food that he is able to, and should, eat, and his likes and dislikes. With physically handicapped patients a knowledge is required of the best and safest position in which to sit them and of the most suitable aids which would assist the patients to feed themselves. The aid of both the speech therapist and physiotherapist can be elicited in this area of care.

(v) Eliminating
In addition to knowing whether the patients are continent or incontinent of urine and/or faeces, it is also important to know whether they suffer from constipation and at what times they tend to eliminate, in order to regulate diets and plan training programmes. The nurse will also need to assess the most suitable clothing for the patients to wear in order to promote continence training.

(vi) Personal cleansing and dressing
The patient's self-help skills in both personal hygiene and dressing can be assessed in association with the occupational therapist, so that there is coordination of training programmes between the ward and O.T. Department, and also so that the O.T. can assess if there is a requirement for any aids that would assist the patient to develop these skills.

(vii) Control of body temperature
This is not concerned only with the nursing of a resident who is suffering from a physical illness. Many nurses for the mentally handicapped fail to meet the every-day needs of their patients in this area. Too frequently they either under- or over-dress them for climate, and where the patients, in particular, are unable to either take excess clothes off, or put extra clothing on, they end up feeling distressed.

Have you ever seen a group of mentally handicapped residents from a hospital on a day trip to the seaside, and immediately known that that was what they were? What was it that made them stick out like a sore thumb?—the fact that they were wearing sweaters and jackets on a nice sunny day.

(viii) Mobilising
Walking defects and the effects of them can be assessed with the help of the physiotherapist and also whether these defects can be either remedied or alleviated through the application of physiotherapy. The physiotherapist can also advise on, and order, the appropriate aids which would assist movement and also advise on the best position in which to place each patient so that movement and rolling is encouraged.

(ix) Working and playing
The assistance of the occupational therapist and psychologist can be sought in order to assess what type of work each patient is capable of and also what type of work would be beneficial to the individual. No patient should be kept back to work in a ward or department because they are useful there when they are capable of better things. Also the patients can be assessed as to what play or leisure activities best suit each patient and what activities would encourage mobility or development.

(x) Expressing sexuality
Whilst assessing whether the patient has the opportunity of mixing with the opposite sex it is

also essential to assess whether they need to be taught how to behave in the company of the opposite sex and whether each patient dresses or is dressed in clothes that are both age and sex appropriate. In this domain it is essential that nurses act as a good rôle model. Assessment will also be needed of the sex educational requirements of each patient and of who would be the best person to instruct them in this area.

(xi) Sleeping

Have the patient's sleeping habits been observed and noted to establish a baseline so that a deviation may be attributed to recent causes?

(xii) Dying

At the appropriate time to be allowed to die with dignity in their familiar surroundings and with those people they know best.

Exercise

As with Orem's model, Roper's may likewise be employed to assess both individual and ward management needs. Work down the column below asking yourself how you meet such needs for yourself. Next, examine how you attempt to enable others to meet these needs while you 'nurse'. Lastly, reflect on how your managerial strategies address these at present.

Maintaining a safe environment
Is the area physically safe? Psychologically safe to try out new relationships? Where do residents perceive the most threat?

Communicating
Do staff communicate professionally or personally about their motives and tensions? Are residents encouraged to share their thoughts, feelings, wishes or desires?

Breathing
Are all staff aware of clients with conditions which affect their breathing? That is epileptic seizures, chronic chest infections or asthma?

Eating and drinking
Are staff aware of food allergies, likes and dislikes of residents? Can residents meet their own needs here when they wish to? If not, why not?

Eliminating
Which residents need dietary help here, or encouragement to exercise? Which training is necessary to induce independence in these areas?

Personal cleansing and dressing
Which garments present which residents with problems? What training is necessary to induce independence in these areas?

Controlling body temperature
What constraints operate to cause residents to stay overdressed upon the ward? Do residents have free access to their own clothes and cooler or warmer areas of the ward?

Mobilising
Are footwear and walking aids available and appropriate to resident needs? Is appropriate physiotherapy being encouraged in those who can benefit from it?

Working and playing
Is play activity planned to enable the development of individual skills? What work activity is most 'self-actualising' for individuals in the area?

Expressing sexuality
What attitudes are demonstrated by staff regarding the client's expressions of sexuality, and how are residents educated to sexual awareness?

Sleeping
Are individual sleep patterns noted and catered for within the area? What happens when a resident wakes up early and would like to make coffee?

Dying
How does the ward culture work through, offer counsel or face up to a resident's death, or the death of a client's family member? Are residents able to be nursed during their last major illness within their own room and near friends?

Personal insights arising from the use of nursing models

It is during the planning stage especially that a nurse may give consideration to the routines and environment of a ward. Can the routine be altered to enrich the meeting of care needs? Or can client grouping be afforded to give more individuality in the overall approach and reduce comparison with a conveyor-belt function?

Planning of care may be drawn up to accommodate both 'long-term' and 'short-term' goal objectives, the short-term plans relating to the immediate attainments possible with the existent resources, and the long-term goals relating to areas where future resources are necessary. Roper's model may therefore supply headings with a regard to future management budgets.

Planning and evaluation go hand in hand, as do short- and long-term goals. If one examines events such as dying, a person's care needs must be planned with regard to short-term comfort—which means an evaluation of his care needs minute-to-minute while also being aware of when to call back his relatives who have expressed the wish to be by his bedside should his condition deteriorate.

Once the specific care and/or training plan has been devised for each individual client, the appropriate care can be given (implemented). It is only when existing data are fully recorded that appropriate care (which includes training) may be given. All too often nurses have been known to say that they 'know their patients so therefore know what care is required by them'. No nurse, however much she knows her patient, is on duty twenty four hours a day, so standards and approaches to care will vary from shift-to-shift, especially when relief staff work on the ward. By recording the plan of care required by an individual, all members of staff are able to refer to the available care plans and thus deliver the appropriate care.

Arguments are often put forward by nurses against nursing models, on the grounds that they are too time-consuming, especially in the area of record-keeping; they often fail to perceive the time to be saved if short-term notes are thorough. For instance, take feeding regimes; if a nurse has not already noted that a client can feed himself solids and fluids—but cannot efficiently steer a spoon from his plate to his mouth—much time might be wasted in feeding him everything before him because a nurse new to the ward doesn't know this information or his level of abilities. Even more frightening, a resident with such skills, if not reinforced may lose them again. Much 'skill-poverty' in mental handicap is induced by nurses ignoring or being unfamiliar with a patient's previous gains. Doing too much for a client is a sure way of wasting time, and much of this can be prevented by effective notes and the recording of nursing observations in the first place. Much useless information is recorded in nursing notes because nurses are not aware of any specific purpose as to why they are writing. Working to a nursing model would help to alleviate this form of wasteful activity also. How useful is the daily recording of 'nil to report', 'went to O.T.' or 'had a quiet night'? Or the six-monthly care review from which nothing new emerges regarding the patient, nursing plan of action or care implementation? We have much to do to put our house in order.

Finding time to do things is endemic in nursing, and serves to discourage the acceptance of the new. Often it is tight routines again at fault here, so that flexibility is lost. Besides, all change need not occur at once; pilot studies might be applied to one or two individuals initially, so that staff develop their skills and adapt to change.

In the field of mental handicap nursing, it is the nursing auxiliaries who, in the majority of hospitals, give most of the direct care to the patients. Thus the more help, encouragement and guidance they receive, the better able they will be to do good work. There is a direct relationship between the help they receive and the quality of care they are able to give.

Supervision of the staff becomes the key to effective leadership, but those in charge must be prepared to change their ideas of what supervision is and consequently their methods of giving it, since the ward sister is concerned with directing the work of the ward team.

Suspicion often surrounds nursing models in that 'they are too high powered' or 'not applicable to us'. The few examples given in this chapter on the care of the mentally handicapped may help nurses to apply their own skills to the benefit of their patient. Nursing models are not high-powered constructions but practical aids. By applying a nursing model to the care of the mentally handicapped, nursing staff will be going in the right direction of applying the philosophy implicit in the 1982 Syllabus of Training: 'They will have the same rights as other people'. Nurses will be ensuring that clients are treated as individuals as opposed to receiving block treatment. When clients receive training 'to care' for themselves, they assume responsibilities and the rights which are frequently denied them. Also it is implicit within the 1982 Syllabus of Training that mentally handicapped people receive services that meet their changing needs; the employment of a nursing model ensures that this will happen.

Mental handicap nursing has traditionally followed in the footsteps of the doctor and assumed an authoritarian approach to care. As Menzies (1961) pointed out

> patients already restricted within the wards have suffered further restrictions through the relationships they have shared with nursing staff. Recipients of care have therefore tended to end up the responsibility of the nurse whose task it is to provide continuous care for patients, day and night, all year round.

As Heath and Law (1982) quoted:

> Frequently nurses are required to co-ordinate the activities of other health care workers and produce appropriate and continuous care of each patient.

In order to do this, nurses must not only be prepared to work in a team, but also encourage the use of a multi-disciplinary approach to care in their own wards. As a team leader, the ward sister is responsible for all nursing care given on her ward and should be concerned with the direction, supervision and evaluation of that care. As part of this responsibility she must coordinate not only the activities of her staff, but also the services of other professional care staff for the benefit of the patients.

At present, the ward report system frequently dominates the tone of the ward. The daily report books act as a managerial monitoring tool, on which are recorded 'incidents'. Examples of the types of incidents which are recorded include: 'Johnny was upset and smashed a window'; 'P.R.N. medication given'; or that 'Lilly appeared unwell'; 'seen by the M.O.'; 'observations to be continued'. It is only following such critical comments that many clients are discussed between the two shifts, and then often in medical terms only. Worse still is the ward report that states there is 'nil to report'—then at the shift hand-over not even one client gets discussed.

The movement away from task-orientated nursing to individual patient care should result in a change from this nonsensical routine between shifts. Each patient may then be discussed at each shift hand-over, and all staff should know about the patients' needs, progresses or regressions. All staff on the ward can then have feelings of involvement.

Nursing has not received much praise for its systems of management. Too frequently nursing management has sought to provide a safe, secure, trouble-free environment. Therapy and individualised care have been little considered in the past. This chapter has illustrated a means of reversing this process.

Critique

The question arises, how appropriate are models of nursing—intended for individualised care—for enquiry at the level of ward management? The more so with a model such as Orem's which tends to discount 'environment' as an entity in itself—preferring to view it as a 'subcomponent of man'.

Depending upon your interpretation of Orem's work, the environment of the ward may be seen as either the least important or most important focus of nursing—the former when taken as a consequence of individual response, the latter when it blocks satisfaction of an individual's needs.

Should a nurse then concentrate upon the development of an individual so that he may affect his environment, or attune to the environment in order to enable greater individual self-care? The author chooses the latter. Orem recognises man and environment as a singular integrated system, and nursing to be a compilation of four types of action influencing this:

(a) judgements as to why patients require nursing;
(b) knowledge of appropriate caring interventions;
(c) educating the patient to self care and greater self-enabling skills; and
(d) adjusting the systems of nursing to meet current circumstances.

The author would seem to have directed her attention to (d) above.

Orem's model has a certain complexity, its breadth makes its simplification even harder; possibly the author may be criticised for reducing its perspective. Conversely, she may be praised for making it the more tangible and practical. The above model generates many more questions than answers, and in this may be seen as creative and opening up further enquiry rather than merely resolving 'problems'.

Roper's work, in contrast, seems readily adaptable to mental handicap care for its activities of living lend themselves to a social educative rôle; then again, its medical bias can limit its appreciation as a tool for social therapy, so no simple answer is evident wherever we look.

Paul Barber

Salient questions

1. How useful is it to apply nursing models to ward management?
2. What insights arise from Orem's work when applied to management, and how do these differ in quality and type from those generated by Roper?
3. Which of the above models is best employed in the mentally handicapped field, and with which clients in particular?

4. How might you make use of this chapter in your own work?

References

General Nursing Council for England and Wales 1982 *Training Syllabus, Register of Nurses, Mental Subnormality Nursing.*

Heath J & Law GM 1982 *Nursing Process—What is it? A Practical Introduction*, NHS Learning Resources Unit, Sheffield.

Henderson V 1966 *The Nature of Nursing. A Definition and its Implication for Practice, Research and Education*, MacMillan Co, New York.

HMSO 1972 *Report of the Committee on Nursing*, Cmnd 5115.

King RD & Raynes NV 1968 An operational measure of inmate management in residential institutions, *Soc. Sci & Med.*, **2**, 41–53.

King RD, Raynes NV & Tizard, J 1971 *Patterns of Residential Care: Sociological Studies in Institutions for Handicapped Children*, Routledge & Kegan Paul, London.

Mayers MC 1972 *A Systematic Approach to a Nursing Care Plan*, Appleton Century Crofts, New York.

Menzies I 1961 *The Functioning of Social Systems as a Defence Against Anxiety*, Tavistock Publications, London.

Nodder Report 1977 *Organisational and Management Problems of Mental Illness Hospitals.* HMSO, London.

Orem D 1980 *Nursing—Concepts of Practice*, McGraw-Hill, New York.

Raynes NV & King RD 1968 *The Measurement of Child Management in Institutions for the Retarded*, Proc. 1st Congress Int. Ass. Sci. Study Ment. Def., Baltimore University Park Press.

Riehl JP & Roy C 1980 *Conceptual Models in Nursing Practice*, Appleton Century Crofts, New York.

Rogers ME 1980 Nursing—A science of unitary man. In: JP Riehl & C Roy (eds), *Models for Nursing Practice*, Appleton Century Crofts, New York.

Roper N *et al* 1983 *Using a Model for Nursing.* Churchill Livingstone, Edinburgh.

Sundeen SJ *et al* 1976 *Nurse–Client Interaction: Implementing the Nursing Process*, The CV Mosby Co, St Louis.

Tizard J 1968 *The Rôle of Social Institutions in the Causation, Prevention and Alleviation of Mental Retardation*, Peabody MIMH, Conference on Socio-Culture Aspects of Mental Handicap, MIMH.

Yura H & Walsh MB 1978 *The Nursing Process*, Appleton Century Crofts, New York.

6

An eclectic model of staff development: supervision techniques to prepare nurses for a process approach— a social perspective

Paul Barber and Ian Norman

Summary

This final chapter underpins everything that has gone before. Using nursing models, the authors contend, is wasted if interpersonal skills and sensitivity are not employed alongside them. Training for these is therefore described. Quality supervision, a concept borrowed from social work, is suggested as helpful in the development of relevant interpersonal clinical skills.

Supervision of a clinical, interpersonal and supportive nature is suggested to enable the provision of 'care for carers'. Supervision is seen as educative and stimulating of therapeutic practice.

Nurture is emphasised rather than managerial control.

Strategies are described to inculcate care skills: learning contracts, peer support, rôle-play, brainstorming and group facilitation.

All these techniques are combined with supervised practice to ensure that nursing models do not fall on professionally shallow ground.

Quality supervision is an educational process when applied to learners, but when applied to patients is taken to be a therapeutic input. In effective supervision education and therapy co-exist for both carer and cared for alike; both disclose their 'humanity' and both grow through the relationship they share.

Paul Barber

Two steps forward and one step backward

The urgency to comply with new fashions of care, be they managerial reorganisation such as the Salmon Report, or fresh clinical approaches like community homes, has historically within the nursing profession driven us to build on weak—or even non-existent—foundations. Hostel care came in before we had come to grips with planning socialisation programmes and long after we had let social aspects of our rôle slip into the hands of play-therapists, voluntary workers and sundry others; a new syllabus of training was foisted upon our learners before their teachers had been prepared accordingly, and now, the philosophy of 'holistic care' has arrived—in the guise of nursing models—while most of the profession still view nursing activity through managerial spectacles.

When staff are improperly prepared for the demands of a 'process-centred' approach—where skill in interpersonal relationships is an essential ingredient of care—they end up performing their nursing in a dutiful manner that reduces the 'social process' to another task, such as talking to a client while they perform procedures upon them. 'Individualised care' then recedes to be replaced by clerical duties such as writing up even more nursing notes. In this climate, routines smother 'process' and the ward remains ensnared at the stage of paying lip-service to models of care.

Nurses in mental handicap are more likely to have been trained in a culture of institutional care, and hence, feel more at ease working in an environment where their rôle is routinely organised. This means that 'change' is often imbued with a good deal of anxiety. In their efforts to retain composure, nurses so conditioned are apt to impose systems of nursing where residents are more managed and controlled than individually cared for.

Nursing process attempts to counteract this by seeking to erase such negative effects as institutional dependence, loss of individuality, isolation and low levels of social skill; these it addresses on the client's behalf, but we tend to forget that similar conditions also blight many nursing staff.

In mental handicap, the nurses' rôle is primarily an educational one. They train, counsel, develop the social and liberate the personal potential of their clients. Knowledge alone is insufficient, so is formal classroom tuition. What they need is on-going professional support so that conflicts may be examined as they arise and relevant on-the-spot skills imparted.

Historically, problems in implementing the nursing process have arisen because clinical supervision has failed to keep pace with new developments in current practice. Many potentially rich influences have evolved: behaviour modification, normalisation, community and hostel provision, self-management schemes and all those interactive features of a process perspective; but the preparation of nurses has failed to keep pace with these changes.

Clinical exposure in handicap nursing has often predominated over a concern for theoretical strategies. 'Experience' was historically seen as something that could not be taught; likewise 'care'. Training schools imparted cognitive data to learners—such as the medical sciences—but left them to reap what practical skills they could from their clinical placements. 'Being a part of the ward team', 'fitting into the institutional culture' and 'being able to quickly

and efficiently complete the work' were major aims of training.

Survival skills versus growth skills

Recently, the concept of quality supervision has acquired educational merit, for growth in patient-centred care has necessitated appraisal of a trainee's 'social competency'. Uniformity of attitude and behaviour—so often sought in the past by service colleagues—is becoming secondary to the sensitive perception of individual need.

Uniformity may have made for ease of management, but we paid the price, for it frustrated initiative and creative adaption (Barber, 1984). The traditional apprenticeship approach to care too often imparted survival skills but left untouched the learner's potential for personal and interpersonal growth. The hospital ran smoothly, people knew where they stood, boundaries were more clearly defined and the nurse did what had to be done, but at a cost, for much was left unquestioned. Analysis of 'what we do and why we do it' is not a strong feature of nursing culture in mental handicap, nor are carers always able to identify what the generative factors are that enrich 'care' and improve 'client conditions and performance'. Because we have left unanalysed what it is that constitutes therapy, custodial frameworks of care have prospered in mental handicap and have been transmitted with more authority than creative therapeutic models. Inertia was allowed to mould the shape of care, for too much energy was required to generate movement, and rejection could ensue from initiating changes to routine systems of work. A little of this is still with us; questioning may still be bred out of nurses by the time of registration—and the survival skills of 'obedience' and 'safety-play' bred in. An orientation to 'safety' may then predominate over other rationales, causing handicapped people to be restricted to uncreative 'oversafe' environments where their development is frustrated and their choices taken from them, and all—some nurses would have us believe—in the interests of their client's own good!

We suggest that efficient and sensitive staff supervision can rectify these faults, for it simultaneously develops the carer while providing a quality control for the service they perform; self-appraisal and rôle-analysis are central to this concept.

A lesson from social work

If we look beyond the bounds of nursing we find that social workers have used a system of qualitative supervision for many years; they have also made use of a 'problem identification and solving approach' to client management akin to the nursing process.

Considerable emphasis is laid in social work upon supervision; it is initiated during early training and—this is where nurses can learn—continued throughout the whole of their career, even to the very top of their profession. We suspect that many nurses view social workers as having a very different rôle to their own; and possibly—in mental handicap—this was a weapon the Jay Report sought to use against them. In reality, both professions share many common features. Both social worker and nurse offer caring interventions, need proficiency in relationship skills, and work from a client-centred, educationally-aware basis. They also share the ethic of public service.

Skills in relationship management are at the heart of successful nursing and social work. Social workers have taken this concept on board and ensured that these skills are acquired via peer support and supervision; nurses by contrast, have failed to 'get their act together' here and, post-registration, have largely to develop themselves.

Caring for carers through quality supervision

'Supervision' often conjures to mind an image of punitive interventions and criticism; we forget that 'processes' may be monitored besides 'tasks' and that nurturing can feature as strongly as critical appraisal. It is useful to remember that counselling has a supervisory aspect also.

With the above qualifications in view, we suggest that supervisors—be they a nurse helping a resident or a charge nurse monitoring a student—should aim to systematically appraise, explore, and analyse just what the care needs of their clients are. To this end, the following observations may usefully guide the performance and planning of supervision:

Supervision has an educational rôle to play
Here the supervisor assumes responsibility for equipping those he supervises with appropriate knowledge and skills.

Supervision has a management rôle
Here the supervisor may evaluate performance, plan and allocate work in the context of the unit and clarify for the learner the aims of the clinical team. The supervisor acts as a managerial culture carrier ensuring that a balance is kept between an individual's level of skill and the nature of work they are assigned.

Supervision needs to provide support
This means a supervisor's approach must recognise the stress that attends the nursing of handicapped people, while trying to reduce the same for client and staff alike. He must be willing therefore to tackle issues causing stress—such as verbal abuse, high noise levels, feelings of anger and frustration and those formal stresses that pressures of bureaucratic management produce. Supervisors must therefore be willing to accept the rôle of advocate. (To ignore stress is to condone it; the short-term hassle of sorting things out is far less debilitating than living with constant unremitting pressure.)

Supervision must stimulate self-aware practice
Reflection and self-evaluation must be reinforced to effect this aim, with the supervisor acting as a catalyst opening up rigid perceptions, thought patterns and responses to re-examination. Here the supervisor works towards the generation of a climate where trust can flourish and confrontation can be safely used.

This is as true for the client as the student; it underpins care—and care is a commodity for everyone.

Modelling counselling and 'awareness' skills via supervision

If we can model skills of caring within supervision, then perhaps these same skills will enter into the nurse–patient relationship. Krikorian and Paulanka (1982) when addressing the question of 'what made for a successful and therapeutic nurse–patient relationship' came to the conclusion that 'self-awareness' was the key to good practice, but that 'interaction' was the catalyst. When describing the training relationship they were caused to observe: 'As the relationship is developing the person is developing.'

The social-exchange process must also occur in supervision, for it reflects so well the caring relationship for which the supervisee is being prepared; it is an essential educational ingredient. The 'client-centred' approach is a far cry from traditional supervisory modes; it is nearer to that climate in which counsellors are trained, where the value of a trusting relationship is the major requisite for the transmission of awareness and empathy (Kagan, 1975; Egan and Cowan, 1979). If a nurse can obtain both personal growth and counselling skills via supervision, then it is possible that much anguish may be removed from nursing's fraught relationships.

A 'caution' we need to note—also from the field of counsellor training—is that supervisors have a tendency to feel more empathy with the supervisee's client than the supervisee themselves (Lambert, 1974). In a profession like nursing where the 'patient' is so often cited as behind all we do, the characteristic of ignoring the worth of junior staff may be even more pronounced.

To summarise our observations so far, ideally, the supervisor should be working towards

—Being more self-aware and explorative of his own responses.
—Trusting of the supervisee and sharing of his thoughts, feelings and perceptions.

—Becoming more open in his intent and acting true to belief and rôle.
—Gaining further experience in counselling and attempting to enhance this skill.
—Being empathetic to his supervisee and less competitive and controlling generally in his relationships with others.

Creating a contract of supervision

'Contracts', in this context, are a negotiated agreement of what the supervisee identifies as his learning needs and what the supervisor has on offer. The aims of supervision, the characteristics of it, techniques to be employed and its time and place are all worked out and put to paper. By this process, the contrasting expectations of supervisor and supervisee are uncovered and—it is to be hoped—resolved.

Figure 6.1 illustrates this process and its outcomes in terms of contractual themes. A supervision contract may also be drawn up for the purpose of staff orientation, clinical instruction, and for the multi-disciplinary team itself; nurse managers, tutors, senior nurses and practitioners working with clients may all make use of 'contracts'. In fact, it is a folly not to do so.

Supervision contracts used with students could be carried from placement to placement. A profile of previous learning and present needs could also be produced; this would ensure continuity between placements. A format is suggested in Figure 6.2. 'Profiles' orientate supervisors to what has gone before and aid recognition of those needs a supervisee brings to the current area. Supervision is not just the prerogative of students—its use is just as relevant to qualified staff. Professional growth is a necessity for all, and we strongly support the use of 'supervision contracts' and 'supervision profiles' for all grades and levels of staff.

Types of supervision

There are essentially two form of supervision: *formal* and *informal*. In the 'formal' type, supervision is the main task; in the 'informal' type, supervision is secondary to the delivery of care.

Fig. 6.1   Creating a supervision contract

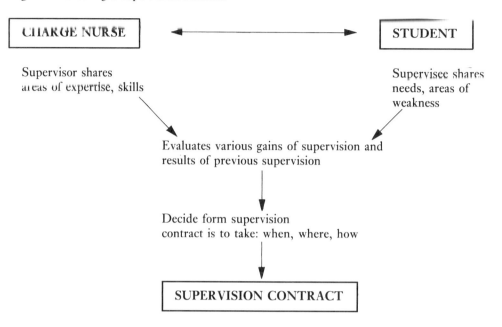

1.	*Types of supervision* Formal or informal, planned or *ad hoc*.
2.	*Techniques of supervision* (a) discussion (b) individualised learning plan (c) problem-solving via group techniques, brain-storming, project work, rôle-play, rôle-reversal, rôle-modelling, etc.
3.	*Supervision arrangements* Time, place, one-to-one or with rest of team.

An example of formal supervision might include a senior nurse and a learner meeting to set learning objectives relating to the clinical area. Informal supervision, conversely, could occur while a senior nurse acts as a rôle model during patient assessment with the student assisting.

In addition to being formal or informal, supervision may be *planned*, as when regular meetings are arranged to occur at weekly intervals; or it may be *ad hoc*, for instance when a crisis occurs upon the ward and consultation and guidance are immediately required and given.

In practice, the difference between formal/informal and planned/*ad hoc* supervision is one of degree rather than kind, distinctions being somewhat blurred. Good supervision is a mix of all the above. A feature of present-day nursing, however, is that most registered nurses have little or no experience of formal/planned supervision and therefore experience difficulty in identifying their supervisory rôle.

Traditionally, formal sessions with trainee nurses are limited to the 'welcome to the ward', halfway interview and final ward report.

Fig. 6.2 Supervision profile

Name David Hawkins		Stage of Training 15th month of training	Date 5/3/87
Check-list of previous gains			**Supervision needs**
Knowledge acquired	Clinical skills	Social skills	
Aware of following models of nursing: Roper; Rogers; Orem; Henderson.	Has assessed patient needs using: Roper; Henderson.	Has interviewed relatives with regard to bereavement.	Needs to look at Peplau's concept of nursing, as this has been recently adopted on units of the hospital to which he is yet to be allocated.
Can discuss genetic conditions and causations with accuracy, in context of factors affecting development prior to birth; and has sufficient skill to teach juniors in this aspect.	Is able to carry out the admission and discharge procedure without guidance.	Relates well to the elderly and infirm.

Handles crises and uncertainty with sufficient composure, working well under stress. | Needs to take greater care in the recording of nursing observations, has a tendency to be dismissive of his rôle in recording data, relying mainly on verbal transmission and the 'good will' of others.

Not clear as to the rôle of trauma in causing mental retardation, nor the various drugs that have been identified with mental handicap. |
| Understands the rationale of community care and normalisation. | Can evaluate his own performance objectively.

Can administer injections (i.m.) | Demonstrates empathy and sensitivity to clients. | Unfamiliar with his responsibilities in regard to compulsory detention via the recent mental health legislation. |
| Knows causation and nursing interventions demanded by following illness states: fever; measles; fractures. | Performs total care—for bed ridden patients— efficiently. | Can counsel 'authoritatively' making use of informative and prescriptive interventions. | Not able to monitor the work of others; knows the theory but says he feels uncomfortable in the supervisory rôle.

Wants to learn more practically about the normalisation process and how it changes existent patterns of care.

Needs more practice in facilitative counselling, especially the use of cathartic and catalytic interventions. |

Qualified staff tend in the main to adopt a predominantly unstructured informal/*ad hoc* style; this is not without risk:

> There is an important difference between making use of informal opportunities arising in the course of a day, and becoming trapped into responding to each and every opportunity as a primary way of working.
>
> (Payne and Scott, 1982)

We believe it is essential that nurses in mental handicap reason through their supervision rôle before it is too late. Changes in practice cannot flower without prior preparation. Unless we make it clear to the national boards that we are doing a better job with our clients than other agencies can do, and can demonstrate a potential to evolve, we may become a lost cause—that is to say, we may lose our right to a separate registration and end up being merely the specialist option of some other care discipline. We believe that the handicapped person would be the greater loser here. Nursing models alone cannot save us, but they can help to liberate the profession's ability to grow and further stimulate this in areas where it is already taking place.

Techniques of supervision

Those same skills we use to plan and contribute to the care of clients may likewise be used for the purpose of staff development; after all, look how similar the process is:

—identification of problematic areas
—planning strategies to address these
—evaluating the outcome of our planned interventions

The supervisory techniques described below provide the 'how' of the above process. Many of the interventions we suggest first saw light in remedial group work, psychotherapy and the educational fields; they are part and parcel of personal growth training and generally share in the common aim of enhancing interpersonal potential.

Identification techniques

(i) Discussion
This forms a major component of most methods, but can differ with regard to being the primary way of working—as in the interview—or a secondary input in such as rôle-play. There is evidence to suggest that retrospective discussion is not as significant a learning tool as many teachers believe, its effect being negligible upon behaviour (Sainsbury, 1980).

A further problem is that group discussions are notoriously difficult to manage. Unshaped dialogue may even enforce negative attitudes and beliefs. Planned agendas and periodic summaries can be helpful in keeping discussions to the point, but skill is required to prevent too rigid a framework inhibiting less confident individuals from expressing their views and feelings. It is useful for the supervisor to remain aware of the range of interventions open to him. The work of Heron (1977) is valuable here as an interactive reference (Figure 6.3).

Too often, conversation can degenerate into a 'time-filler', a social pleasantry or 'stimulus response'. Heron's intervention analysis helps us avoid these blind alleys. We can now examine our own style and 'plan' our contributions. It may seem novel to plan conversation, but defining the intention offers a certain clarity. Just examine the prospective use. The first three (authoritative) interventions (prescriptive; informative; confronting) are valuable in setting the formal framework of supervision; the second (facilitative) set (cathartic; catalytic; supportive) solicit responses from the supervisee; both styles are client-centred in their approach, and both—though directed to differing concerns—when sensitively used are therapeutic. Successful supervision makes relevant use of all six interventions. Encouraging the subject for supervision to be aware of six-category intervention analysis is a most worthwhile assignment in itself.

(ii) Projects
These may be used fruitfully to assess the needs of individual clients or patient groups. Various approaches—as suggested by specific models of

Fig. 6.3 Heron's six-category intervention analysis

Authoritative

1. *Prescriptive*: Give advice, be judgemental/critical/evaluative. A prescriptive intervention is one that explicitly seeks to direct the behaviour of the client, especially though not exclusively, behaviour that is outside or beyond the practitioner–client interaction.

2. *Informative*: Be didactic, instruct/inform, interpret. An informative intervention seeks to impart new knowledge and information to the client.

3. *Confronting*: Be challenging, give direct feedback. A confronting intervention directly challenges the restrictive attitude/belief/behaviour of the client.

Facilitative

4. *Cathartic*: Release tensions, encourage laughter/crying. A cathartic intervention seeks to enable the client to experience painful emotion.

5. *Catalytic*: Be reflective, encourage self-directed problem-solving, elicit information. A catalytic intervention seeks to enable the client to learn and develop by self-direction and self-discovery within the context of the practitioner–client situation, but also beyond it.

6. *Supportive*: Be approving, confirming, validating. A supportive intervention affirms the worth and value of the client.

nursing—could be employed and the respective benefits of one or more models contrasted and discussed.

(iii) On-the-job assessment
Though reminiscent of nursing in its pre-nursing process era, this has the advantage of immediate feed-back. Client needs and the necessary nursing skills a student may require are readily observable in the dynamics of nursing activity. To enrich on-the-job identification of potential need states, pre-activity and post-activity evaluation sessions need to be planned, the former for examining the aims of action, the latter to evaluate how well these were met.

Planning strategies

These aim to structure supervisory encounters so that sessions are purposeful to all concerned; in fact, nursing models of care are themselves examples of planning techniques!

(i) Self-directed learning contracts
An example of this is shown in Figure 6.4. The supervisees, be they a client or student, set their own learning objectives and devise methods to meet these. Senior students are more able—in our experience—to use this method in its pure 'self-directed' form; juniors tend to need initial guidance.

(ii) Brain-storming
Though applicable at most stages, brain-storming is especially potent in breaking away from routine solutions and exploring creative ventures when other tried-and-tested methods have failed. Ideas, no matter how bizarre, are recorded upon a sheet of paper without comment or criticism, later being sifted through in reflective discussion. This technique can be fun when used sparingly, but may become tedious if over-used.

Rehearsing social strategies

(i) Rôle-play
This may be performed by the supervisor playing a client, while the supervisee tries out a planned intervention or suitable care strategy. This technique is of crucial importance in social skill training, e.g. learning to tolerate uncertainty,

Fig. 6.4   Learning contract

Name Teresa Martin	**Placement** Beech Ward	**Date** 26/5/87	

(a) What do you see as your key learning objectives for this clinical placement? (Write these below.)

(b) What help or guidance do you think you require to achieve the above objectives? (Identify people, libraries etc., who can help you.)

(c) How will you evaluate your learning? (Who may assist you here; can client feed-back be used or peer evaluation?)

(d) What new insights have arisen from this exercise to take with you for future use?

facing up to rejection or dealing with simulated crises situations.

(ii) Rôle-reversal
Here the supervisor may swap his rôle with that of his student to allow the latter to develop his own supervisory skills. It may likewise be performed when a supervisor and supervisee find themselves antagonistic towards each other or locked in futile win-or-lose dynamics where negative 'game-play' necessitates resolution. An over-defensive student may, in presenting the supervisor's case, come to see in a new objective light the underlying conflicts and problems, but devoid of the need to defend his personal view, so escaping emotional entanglement.

Review/evaluation techniques

(i) Nominal group review
A clinical team may be asked to evaluate the effect of the introduction of a process model upon the ward. Individuals would first be asked to work alone and silently upon the issue. After a predetermined time, ideas and observations are shared. Voting is employed to resolve disagreements. The particular advantage of this method is that all staff—regardless of rank or personal assertiveness—may offer contribution and involvement.

(ii) Questionnaire
Open-ended questions soliciting answers to such statements as:

What do you most like about . . . .?
What do you least like about . . . .?
How would you improve upon . . . .?

Methods such as these tend to be coolly received initially—because of their newness and their demand of response—they don't let you turn off and dismiss them as easily as conventional practices—but if persevered with they solicit greater commitment.

Supervision arrangements

These are alternatives to planned/*ad hoc*, and formal/informal modes. Regular planned supervision is relevant when both participants share in a common work area but in situations where distances are involved, time is short or specialist training is required, alternative arrangements are necessary.

(i) Pair supervision
Two experienced nurses meet to regularly share problems, offer consultation and counsel.

(ii) Peer group support
Groups of staff meet to give mutual support and explore the issues that affect them.

(iii) Facilitated groups
These usually have a training function, an experienced facilitator enabling the examination of sensitive material, emotional conflicts or just releasing safely the pressures of everyday caring. Facilitated groups may be commenced prior to 'peer support groups' to establish stable dynamics or a climate for future work. Here feelings are supervised rather than tasks.

Conclusion

This chapter has sought to outline the options available in supervision. Its bias is in its belief that models of nursing will not grow, nor be of any use whatsoever, until quality supervision has been established and training in the social skills described in this work implemented for clients and carers alike.

> *It is wisdom to know others; it is enlightenment to know oneself.*
> (Lao-tzu, 5th Century B.C.)

References

Barber P 1984 A radical view of nursing uniforms, *Nursing Standard*, 29th November.

Egan G & Cowan M 1979 *People in Systems: A Model of Development in the Human Service Professions and Education*, Brooks & Cole, California.
Heron J 1977 *Behaviour Analysis in Education and Training*, Human Potential Research Project, University of Surrey.
Jay Committee 1979 *Report of the Committee into Mental Handicapped Nursing Care*, DHSS, London.
Kagan N 1975 Influencing human interaction—eleven years with IPR, *Canadian Counsellor*, 9, 74-97.
Krikorian D & Paulanka B 1982 Self-awareness—the key to a successful nurse patient relationship? *Journal of Psychiatric Nursing & Mental Health Services*, 20, 6.
Lambert M 1974 Supervisory and counselling process: a comparative study, *Counsellor Education and Supervision*, 14, 54-60.
Menzies I 1961 *The Functioning of Social Systems as a Defence Against Anxiety*. Tavistock Publications, London.
Payne C & Scott T 1982 *Developing Supervision of Teams in Field and Residential Social Work*, National Institute for Social Work.
Sainsbury E 1980 Client need, social work method and agency function—a research perspective, *Social Work Service*, 23.

Epilogue

Mental handicap nursing is at a crossroads; the medical model—so long with us—is waning in power, community care is in the ascent, and client involvement and advocacy are influences that demand assimilation. Nursing models may help us here because they involve clients, facilitate negotiation and encourage rôle analysis. But nurses themselves need preparation if they are to capitalise on these benefits.

Facilitation skills, educational inputs and improved qualitative supervision have been suggested as essential prerequisites if nurses are to make successful use of nursing models. Otherwise, nurses may end up clerking their observations in new ways while performing in the same old ones.

Nurses, from the evidence of this work, are beginning to put their house in order; if they are withdrawn from mental handicap, as might be the case if movement to the community outpaces the preparation of community nurses, mentally handicapped people will suffer. The social services are ill-prepared for the high dependency and specialist requirements of a mentally handicapped population. Nurses have learned from their mistakes; social workers still have their mistakes to make with the client group in question.

The authors of this book believe it is in the interests of care that nurses synthesise the skills of social workers, educationalists, and counsellors, so that they may fully achieve the status of 'therapists'. There is really no other choice; if we fail to do this we become superfluous, and a hotelier service can be performed by anyone.

Paul Barber

Index